Mindful Movement

Mastering Your Hidden Energy

D1570912

Also by Sang H. Kim

Vital Point Strikes

Power Breathing

Ultimate Flexibility

Ultimate Fitness Through Martial Arts

The Art of Harmony

Teaching Martial Arts: The Way of The Master

1,001 Ways To Motivate Yourself & Others

Martial Arts After 40

Complete Taekwondo Poomsae

Muye Dobo Tongji: The Comprehensive Illustrated Manual of Martial Arts of Ancient Korea

Mindful Movement

Mastering Your Hidden Energy

Sang H. Kim, Ph.D.

Turtle Press • Washington DC

To contact the author or to order additional copies of this book:
Turtle Press
500 N. Washington St #1545
Rockville MD 20849
www.TurtlePress.com

LCCN: 2013033833
ISBN: 978-1-938585-28-9

Printed in the United States of America

The Turtle Press name and logo are trademarks of Turtle Press.

Warning-Disclaimer: This book is designed to provide information on specific
skills used in health and fitness. You are urged to read all available material,
learn as much as you wish about the subjects covered in this book and tailor the
information to your individual needs. Anyone practicing the skills presented in
this book should be physically capable to do so and have the permission of a li-
censed physician before participating in this activity. Every effort has been made
to make this book as complete and accurate as possible. However, there may be
mistakes, both typographical and in content. The author, publisher, printer and
distributors shall neither have liability nor responsibility to any person or entity
with respect to loss or damages caused, or alleged to have been caused, directly or
indirectly, by the information contained in this book.

Library of Congress Cataloguing in Publication Data

Kim, Sang H., author.
  Mindful movement : mastering your hidden energy / Sang H. Kim, Ph.D.
     pages cm
  Includes index.
  ISBN 978-1-938585-28-9
  1. Breathing exercises. 2. Mind and body. I. Title.
  RA782.K56 2013
  613'.192--dc23
                              2013033833

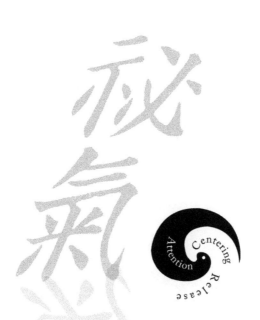

*...hidden yet always working, being
present everywhere yet found nowhere...*

Contents

ROAD MAP

Author's Note

1. MINDFULNESS | 11
3-Step Mindful Practice | 13
Interoception | 16
Balance Within | 17
About Meditation | 19
Benefits of Mindfulness | 21
How to Practice Meditation in Brief | 23

2. MINDFUL MOVEMENT | 25
Attention | 27
Centering | 30
Release | 32

3. MBX-12 | 35
A Brief Overview of MBX-12 | 36
The Basics | 38
Self-Assessment | 42
Connecting the Flow | 43
MBX-1: Awakening | 42
Mindful Practice | 49
Deep Breathing Methodology | 50
The Mechanics of Breathing | 51
Breathing Techniques | 52
MBX-2: Carrier | 54
Ki: Inner Energy | 58
Reception of Energy | 59
Inviting Ki In | 60
Balancing Yin and Yang Energy | 61
How Does Ki Work? | 63
Energy Centers | 65
MBX-3: Infinity | 66
Twisting the Limbs | 70

MBX-4: Finger Wheels | 72
   Selective Senses | 76
   Circadian Impacts | 77
   Fluidity of Movement | 78
   Calming the Nerves | 79
MBX-5: Peacock | 80
   Impact on Circulation | 84
   Blood Follows Ki | 85
MBX-6: Twins | 86
   Stress Resilience | 90
MBX-7: Big Bow | 92
   Proprioception | 96
   Change Your Mood | 97
MBX-8: Lotus | 98
   Ki Energy Paths | 102
MBX-9: Condensing | 104
   Invisible Precedes Visible | 109
   Explosive Energy | 110
   Nasal Breathing | 112
   The Importance of NO and CO_2 | 113
MBX-10: Planting | 114
   Triple Warmer: Virtual Organ | 118
   Oxygen Equals Energy | 119
   Breath Control | 120
MBX-11: Cradling | 122
   Mind-Body Unity | 127
   Stress Buffering | 128
   Sleep Breathing | 129
MBX-12: Unity | 130
MBX-12 SEQUENCE | 134

4. MBX MUDRA | 140

5. WELLNESS APPLICATIONS | 157

6. CONCLUSION | 178

Meet the Author | 179

Index | 181

Road Map

The goal of MBX, mindful movement and deep breathing exercises, is to invigorate your inner energy flow by activating *the four pillars of energy transformation*: mindfulness, movement, breath, and meridians.

The first and second pillars are explained in Chapters 1: Mindfulness and Chapter 2: Mindful Movement. The last two pillars and the twelve MBX postures presented in this book (MBX-12) are explained in detail in Chapter 3. Each posture section includes an introduction to the posture, step-by-step practice guidance, focal points, self-assessment criteria, meridian chart, expected effects, focal point illustration, and short essays to help you deepen your understanding of MBX principles and the underlying mechanisms. You can also view a video demonstration of all 12 postures at Youtube (http://www.youtube.com/watch?v=kWE-m6uQOxo).

Chapter 4 includes 13 MBX Mudras, symbolic hand movements with practical functions. Each mudra activates meridians in the hand and affects energy flow in the corresponding organ(s). Mudras are a good way to practice mindfulness when you cannot do full body exercise such as MBX-12. Chapter 5 has wellness applications of MBX postures that can help you relieve anxiety or stress-related headaches and improve balance.

The text topics located between the exercises are not meant to be read sequentially. Instead, browse through them and read the ones appeal to you at the time. As you advance, you will find that different sections have more meaning for you. Reading the first two chapters before you begin to practice is highly recommended. They will help you understand the fundamental concepts of mindfulness and mindful movement.

Author's Note

For beginners, this book may be hard to grasp initially. The postures that make up the core of MBX (mindful movement and deep breathing exercises) integrate *the four pillars of energy transformation*: mindfulness, movement, breath, and meridians.

If you have experience with practicing one or more of the four pillars, that will form your foundation for understanding MBX. If not, start from the basics and learn one movement at a time. Once you understand one posture well, you can apply the same principles to practicing subsequent postures. The more you practice, the more you will come to integrate the four pillars without conscious effort and achieve a flow experience where all become one.

As you learn the postures and practice methods, it is important to follow directions, practice each posture mindfully, feel the flow, and integrate it into your body's natural character.

For advanced practitioners, the goal is to attain *oneness of the four pillars*. MBX integrates your moving body with your breath, redirects energy flow along the 12 meridians, and unites the mind with all in the present.

1
Mindfulness

Mindfulness, *the first pillar of energy transformation*, is bringing deliberate attention to the present moment without judgment. The objective of being mindful is to connect the mind with the body. As human beings, we are not always conscious of our bodies. Most of time, we are just busy with the business of life.

Is being mindful hard to practice? Yes and no.

Yes, because we forget things. We live purposefully and without purpose. We are used to being judgmental in literally every area of our lives. And we must. Without judgment, we can be vulnerable.

No, because we can be mindful by simply paying attention to what we think and do. Being mindful does not mean we should be vigilant at all times. Indeed, quite the opposite is true. We can be simply aware of what we think and do.

The ultimate experience of being mindful occurs when we forget about everything, even the mindful self and doing. In that mode we are full of energy, utterly self-generated. Hence mindfulness is *the first pillar of energy transformation*. However, a paradox is that to be mindful, one must not try to be mindful, and to not be mindful, one must be mindful.

Can we cut it short? The answer is yes. We can skip the mindful part. How? By just doing what we like to do when we feel like doing it, in the way we feel the best. No thought, no mind. It's a vacation of the mind, so to speak. You kick the mindful thing out of the equation from the start.

Total physical immersion with mental emptiness. Just doing.

For most of us, this is quite a challenge. As in rock climbing, where we use a niche to securely place a foot or fingers, we need somewhere tangible to place our mind. Having something to think about or focus on keeps us oriented. It anchors the mind to a specific moment in time, preventing it from fleeting. It keeps our awareness contained within our body so that the body does not do things randomly.

Once the mind is contained, the body can fly. When the body is in motion, the action generates an even greater amount of energy. Thus movement is *the second pillar of energy transformation* (discussed in Chapter 2: Mindful Movement).

The niche the mind can grab is *interest* which holds your attention. In this book, we use the body as the target of interest to contain the mind. For example, your hand. When you stretch your fingers wide open, your mind comes to your hands. Instantly.

The body is amazing. We think the mind is the master of us. But I often think the opposite is true. The mind is quite impatient and radical in action, hard to herd. But when the body moves, the mind comes along. Physical actions generate mental engagement.

When our body moves in flow-like motion, as in dancing, the body merges with the rhythm. The mind tunes in, and the body contains the mind. They dance together, paying attention to each other.

The practice of being mindful begins with a small step. Bring your awareness back to you and your actions. Let it stay there. For example, when you eat, be aware of chewing slowly and tasting the food. When you walk, be aware of your posture. When you sit, keep your spine straight. Doing so gives you strength and room for breath. Press the diaphragm slightly downward toward the belly. This helps your body and mind come into focus and equanimity. By paying attention to small things in the way you act and think, you can lift yourself to the next level. Amuse yourself. Let yourself grow.

Unless you can totally lower your guard, struggles are inevitable. To lessen struggles, practice no holding, no pushing, and no pulling. Allow your mind to be free. Just point your mind to where to stay. Then guide it on an expedition through your actions. Mindful movement just does that.

Let the mind lose itself in the course of mindful movement. And let the movement and mind merge through breath, a unification of *the first, second, and third pillars of energy transformation*. Your breath connects your body and mind. When the connection grows stronger, let it go. All that is left is an emptiness of the mind, the mind that holds nothing but the experience itself. The more you practice, the more you can empty yourself. The more you can empty your mind, the lighter you feel. The void then is filled with essential energy which flows through the 12 meridians, *the fourth pillar of energy transformation*.

This way, moment-to-moment struggles vanish and a sprout of wisdom emerges. It's the beginning of a small revolution within. It's an amazing experience called *mindfulness*.

3-STEP MINDFUL PRACTICE

To experience mindfulness in MBX practice, be aware of the *mental component* of each posture, focusing on *attention, centering*, and *release*.

Attention should be *intentionally* focused on a part of your body. The mind tends to wander around everywhere but the present, often settling more on regrets of the past or planning for the future. But the body is stuck here and now. So we bring the mind to the body as a way of anchoring it. For example, by paying attention *visually and physically* to the middle of your open hand, you can contain your mind to here and now.

Centering means *intentionally* creating a physical posture and mental space in which you feel strong and competent. You direct your inner energy to the place where you want it to be. Typically these places are somewhere in the middle of your body (page 65): the lower belly area (also known as the lower energy center) for developing physical energy and the chest area (also known as the middle energy center) for developing mental awareness. If you are overstimulated, bring your energy down. If you feel low, bring the energy up. You can control your energy levels by physically lowering your posture or by regulating your breath. For example, deep breathing while in the Infinity Posture (see page 66 for details) can be calming.

Release is *intentionally* stepping back from and disengaging with your thoughts, emptying the mind. Let things go, but accept and embrace what's left: your body, the container of your thoughts and feelings. This is an unburdening and refreshing stage.

Three-step mindful practice is a process for guiding your physical and mental energy. Energy is transient. It changes. It is consumed and built. It is discharged and recharged. With your intention, when you are attentive, centered, and letting go, somewhere deep within you, fresh energy rises. It is a seed for growth and strength. You can develop it for an inner revolution in you. It enlightens you.

But, how do we really do it? Here is what I have found useful: **First, notice what is happening in your body.** If you have *pain*, where is it coming from? Change the position of your body so that you can relax that particular area and ease the pain. Then bring your *attention* to the opposite side of the body, like using a crutch to support an injured leg. Imagine that opposite side is your inner ally, supporting the painful side.

The second step is to recognize what is on your mind. Recognize the most troubling *thought* which you cannot stop from recurring or arising. Recognize its pattern. Is it from inside you or from outside? Does it make you angry, frustrated, depressed, worried, or afraid? Be aware of what it is and where it may have come from, but leave it alone.

By being aware but leaving it alone, you practice the *centering* principle, a way of neutralizing the negative effect and establishing your leverage to heal. At this stage, you may practice an MBX posture of your choice to activate the relevant meridians for alleviating your discomfort. *The MBX posture is a venue for you to engage your body with your consciousness.* While your body is participating in physical movement, your mind follows your actions, observing the changes in your body. As part of this process, your mind may overreact to your pain or troubling thoughts. Be open to whatever arises. You don't need to stop this hyperactive reaction of the mind. Let it be as best you can.

The third step is to accept that feelings and thoughts are transient. Also remember that the transient transits from one form to another. Allow them to be within the space that you are monitoring. They will leave soon. The more you try to turn them off, the longer they linger. Allow your feelings and thoughts some freedom to passively stay as your body's guest for a while. Then, allow them to transit to somewhere else. While you wait for them to prepare to take their leave, ask your troubling thoughts, 'What are you?', 'Where are you from?', 'Why are you here?', 'What can I do for you?' Getting to know them and specifically itemizing them without any attachment to their negative effect will help you better understand what you are suffering from and why. Then, practice *letting go.*

Throughout these stages, be fully mindful in your doing without distraction (even without thinking about overcoming your pain or troubling thoughts). You will outdo your expectation. You will become a diligent doer while vigilantly observing your problems.

---

3 STEP MINDFUL PRACTICE

---

1. Attention

2. Centering

3. Release

INTEROCEPTION

Interoception is our internal sense of the physiological condition of the body. It includes all of our internal physical sensations including pain, temperature, hunger, thirst, breathlessness, and other sensations that originate in our organs and muscles.

Simply, it is how we feel. More formally, it is called body awareness. Interoception is important because how we feel dictates our actions. Feelings from the body motivate our behavior.

Thoughts can mask the condition of the body, but feelings directly reflect what is going on in our body. Therefore, feeling is a more reliable source for assessing whether the body is in homeostasis, a stable internal condition.

Our awareness of feelings from the body conveys information about the physiological conditions of the particular organs and tissues. Is this sensation painful or pleasurable? Accordingly, we act. We seek help when we are in pain. We continue an activity when it is pleasurable. Feelings motivate actions.

Feeling and motivation are the essence of emotion. Under the influence of positive emotion, we nourish a positive inner environment; under negative emotion, we consume inner resources and burn a great deal of energy, often for unproductive outcomes.

Why is interoception important?

Because it conserves energy. Energy efficiency is the core value of homeostasis, the result of centuries of biological evolution. It is the primary purpose of our awareness.

For energy efficiency, the communication between the body and brain needs to flow without disruption. The body should send clear and correct signals. The brain should be noise-free to accept the information without interference and interpret it correctly. When this occurs, our emotional feeling is balanced and the resulting action is appropriate and supports physical and mental homeostasis.

Interoception coincides with the underlying meaning of mindfulness. Mindfulness is paying attention on purpose in the present moment and connecting the mind with the body non-judgmentally. Openness and acceptance are the foundation of mindfulness and of interoception. The effects of how we perceive and feel are significant to how the body behaves. If the brain perceives a false alarm as real, the body instantly prepares to fight or flee. If the perception is filtered and the brain discerns the false alarm, the body maintains homeostasis.

By practicing body awareness, by tuning in to and becoming aware of your interoceptive sensations, you can improve how you listen to what your body says and connect it to your brain, free of interference. This can be a way to attain peace of mind and reduce the stress of not knowing where the real threat lies. It is seeing the problem and designing the steps to solve it by just asking the body, "How do you feel?"

Interoception is an innate intelligence, like having many brains spread out all over in the body. Being tuned in to your interoceptive sensations is central to stopping the body's tendency to default to autopilot responses, which are often unhealthy and habitual.

BALANCE WITHIN

The mind-body battle occurs when your mind wants to be in tranquility but your body can't be still, or your body needs some rest but your mind keeps racing. Job stress, family obligations, ambition for success, financial distress, or obsessive worry about any of dozens of other things drives us to discord of the mind and body.

For the health and happiness of ourselves and our loved ones, we need to choose to stop the cycle of discord. We need to strive for the ideal balance: achieving tranquility in the midst of our busy life and reclaiming a dynamic lifestyle amidst sedentary modern life patterns.

Attainment of inner stability of the mind and body has been a timeless assignment given to human beings. Hundred of years ago, Walter Cannon, of Harvard Medical School, coined the term 'homeostasis' to describe what the body tries to do in response to changes thrust upon us in order to maintain our inner balance.

If everything were constant and predictable, it would be easy for us to achieve inner stability and master our body, thus achieving true homeostasis. Our reality, however, is constantly changing. There are too many variables for us to even know, let alone control.

The old paradigm of homeostasis suggested that we may be able to rule over our reality. Yet, homeostasis cannot account for the unpredictable nature of our internal and external environments. A new paradigm, however, states that we do not and cannot know all of the variables of our reality. The new model, called 'allostasis', proposes that we maintain stability through change rather than through a constant state of sameness. Allostasis encompasses all of the actively adaptive mechanisms of the body in response to stressors that are both predictable and unpredictable.

There is, however, a cost to allostasis, which is termed *allostatic overload*[1]. The adaptive processes of allostasis involve the production of adrenalin, cortisol and other chemical mediators. These chemical messengers help the body adapt to acute stressors in the short-term. When stressors are prolonged, allostatic overload occurs, resulting in "wear and tear" on the body and brain.

Ironically, allostatic overload can result from both insufficient energy to meet the body's demands or an excess of energy for the body's current needs. In both cases, abnormal physiologic changes occur. Ultimately, the chronic presence of allostatic load can lead to the development of hypertension, diabetes, obesity, and various mental illnesses.

The good news is that in the allostatic model, occasionally encountering unusual or never-before-seen variables is not seen as a failure of the body to maintain homeostasis (as it was in the old model), but rather a healthy response to predictive fluctuations. To cope with a changing environment at every level, the body needs

---

1   Coined by Bruce S. McEwen, Ph.D. Alfred E. Mirsky Professor, Rockefeller University.

to respond to internal and external cues simultaneously from the minute adjustment of hormonal levels to the synchronization of our biorhythm to diurnal and seasonal cycles.

Considering the enormous magnitude of the work our body must do to sustain optimal health, it is important that we understand the larger picture of how the mind and body are integrated. Rather than seeing allostasis as a low-level physiologic mechanism, we should consider the powerful capacity of allostatic adaptation for restoration of the body as an organic whole. The essential goal of allostasis is regaining the balance within the body and optimizing our global well-being via thousands of minute adjustments, many too small for us to even notice.

Like the yin-yang diagram in which two opposing elements act independently yet interdependently for the harmony of the whole, our mind and body reciprocally act together and react against each other. In this way, they constantly seek to restore balance within the body as well as a natural accord with the outer environment.

ABOUT MEDITATION

The heart of meditation lies in self-initiated purpose, self-directed attention, and self-fulfilled commitment. The mind is cyclic in nature, constantly changing its form and place from a simple idea here to a multiplicity of the wildest dreams over there.

It is natural that the mind drifts from one moment to another, from a less attention-grabbing event to stronger stimuli. Overwhelming stresses often engulf the mind and the mind becomes the stressor itself, resulting in it becoming an unintended victim of the vicious cycle of negativity. Out of control, the freely moving mind becomes problematic, consuming enormous amounts of energy and causing stress.

Meditation is a method to restrain the wildness of the mind and restore its original nature. It is a vehicle that facilitates a balanced inner environment and develops the state of being mindful by creating emotional and mental space within yourself.

Breathing, *the third pillar of energy transformation* (pages 50-53), plays a crucial role in creating this internal space, calming the mind and shifting the attention from the stressor to more simple, manageable bodily sensations. This breathing-induced shift in attention creates distance from your feelings toward the stressor.

As long as you maintain your attention on the process of breathing and meditation, in time, changes occur in your awareness. You will develop a deepening insight into what you have been struggling with as you move away from being a participant in the stressful events to becoming an objective observer. Once this happens, you may be able to observe your thoughts from a different perspective. This prevents you from getting caught in the vicious cycle of negative thoughts resulting in an increased reservoir of inner energy.

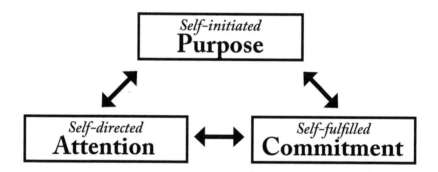

The heart of mindful meditation consists of three axioms: purpose, attention, and commitment. They are not separate components but one in nature. When you have purpose, you will pay attention and be committed. The three are different aspects of a single process of being mindful.

When it comes to shifting your perspective, interoception has a great influence. Interoception is an inner awareness of your physical condition. It is about *how you feel*. Feelings from the body motivate your behavior because feelings directly reflect what is going on in your body. On the contrary, thoughts often mask the real condition of the body. That is why, in meditation, ritualistic physical postures and movements are used for regulating the mind.

Meditation is a *passive* process of accepting yourself as you are without judgment. Can you accept your thoughts and feelings as they are, without judgement? Not an easy task in theory. But a natural accomplishment in actuality. Because the moment you accept the passivity and choose to do so, it no longer is a passive reception, but rather an active engagement with yourself—an ideal self or a larger self. In this mental state, the space within you grows infinitely.

Paradoxically, you begin to regulate your thoughts and feelings without actual regulation. You enter a flow state. Introspective awareness increases and physical sensations decrease. Your focus shifts from physical and emotional stresses to a new inner environment that is stress resilient.

BENEFITS OF MINDFULNESS

Being mindful of the body's movement helps us concentrate on what we are doing in the present moment. By containing the mind in the body, it reduces our tendency to be distracted. Because of the focus on a specific target, the mind wanders less. The brain utilizes its resources to its full innate efficiency.

Efficient brain function naturally results in less burden to the body. Physical distress lessens; the mood evens out; and emotional control resumes. These positive changes are linked to a reduction of pain sensitivity as well.

The practice of localizing attention to the body, in fact, increases sensory information in the brain. As the amount of sensory information flowing from the body to the brain increases, the activity of the cortex in the brain increases. This further enhances cellular communication between the body and the brain. The closer body-brain connection is a key element for heightening our awareness.

A greater awareness of our body and mind underlies the therapeutic benefits of mindfulness. Consider that as an organism, we have a tendency to reorganize ourselves as a whole when we experience loss. We adapt to change, the loss. We process the information of the loss and emerge with a new self as a result of the communication between the body and brain. It is innate, natural, and organic. This is the very definition of stress resilience.

In summary, we undergo constant self-therapy as an adaptation, progressing towards our greater self, the embodiment of the unity between the body and mind.

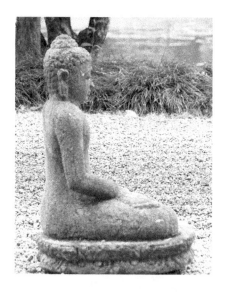

The term 'essential energy' is used in many Eastern cultures. It is known as chi in China, prana in India, lung in Tibet, and ki in Korea and Japan. Traditionally, the concept of energy has been an important component in various medicinal approaches, including Chinese and Korean medicine and Indian Ayurveda.

How to Practice Meditation in Brief

Make a Choice

1. Decide on a place and time for your meditation.
2. Decide the duration of the session. You may begin with as little as one minute.
3. Gradually increase the length of sessions according to your comfort level.
4. End each session on a positive note.

Find Your Posture

1. Sit on a blanket or mat.
2. Bring your feet in front.
3. Try many ways of arranging your feet to find what works best for you. For example, cross your legs with one ankle over the other.
4. Erect your spine and neck.
5. Rest your wrists on the inner bones of the knees.
6. Relax your shoulders.
7. Put your chin slightly down. Relax your facial muscles.
8. Press the diaphragm slightly toward the belly for heightened awareness.

Focus

1. Fix your eyes on one spot in front of you.
2. Breathe slowly through your nose.
3. Sit for a minute, focusing on breathing.
4. Keep inhalation and exhalation even in duration at first.
5. Gradually make exhalation longer than inhalation.
6. As you progress, expand the breathing cycle (5, 10, 15 seconds per breath).

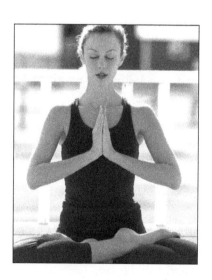

Shift in Perspective

During meditation, mentally step back and disengage yourself from your thoughts.

Shift your attention to your inhalation and exhalation.

Be purposeful in your activity.

Pay attention to your breathing.

Be committed.

2

Mindful Movement

MBX aims at cultivating the flow of inner energy, which is the essence of our life force. There are three principles for practice: *attention, centering, and release.* Each of these principles has a specific *physical component* in MBX practice. By translating the conceptual principles into physical practice, we make them easier to attain.

The *Attention* component brings the eyes to focus on a specific part of the body (e.g., the center of the palm while stretching your fingers) reducing distractions caused by external sensory stimuli and allowing the mind to feel internal sensations, guided by visual attention.

The *Centering* component brings the physical body lower than usual, allowing us to feel the force of gravity and changes in the inner energy dynamics of the lower limbs. By sinking the body lower, we encourage our inner force to rise from the feet, traveling upward to the thigh, stomach, chest, and to the brain. Centering enhances our sense of balance, increases inner strength, and helps to strengthen sense of self.

The *Release* component works like emptying a cup so that it can be filled anew. Using a long mindful exhalation is a cleansing process, expelling carbon dioxide to allow for inhaling fresh oxygen. Releasing also triggers a mental letting go. By practicing letting go, the body naturally takes in more energy.

A full circle of **Attention-Centering-Release** is a seamless proactive process of influx, diffusion and efflux, cleansing the body of stale energy and taking in fresh energy. This process, constituting *the second pillar of energy transformation*, is healing and energizing, not only at the cellular level, but in the systemic and holistic dimension. Through the practice of MBX, the mind and body become an integrated whole, communicating reciprocally for optimal internal balance.

Yin Yang in Brief

Yin and yang are two opposing yet complimentary forces in the universe. Ki, the essential inner vital energy, resides simultaneously in both yin and yang, yet ki itself is neither yin nor yang. Ki is a neutral base substance that is present in all beings.

Lao Tzu, the founder of Taoism, described Ki as an energy hidden yet always working, being present everywhere yet found nowhere. The true nature of yin and yang is constant change. Through attraction and repulsion the balance between both energy forms infinitely fluctuates in multiple dimensions.

There are two types of ki: expressive and receptive ki. Expressive ki is yang-type which presents outside of the body. Receptive ki is yin-type which radiates inside of you. The two types of ki flow after our consciousness, thoughts, intention, and will. When expressed, ki of the sender connects with ki of the receiver causing arousal of new consciousness. If both ki flows match, positive changes may occur. Conversely, ill-matched ki may result in negative outcomes.

3 Step Mindful Movement

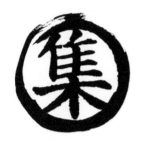

ATTENTION

Attention is an active awareness of and engagement with the world around and inside of us. Our attention can be directed narrowly to a small object or can be broadly spread out to the vastness of our surroundings. Attention may be brought to a passing train, a flying bee, the smell from your kitchen, the music on the radio, your back pain, a friend's wedding, a bill that needs paying, a car accident, your weight, sleep problems, a promotion, your children...

The quality of your attention affects the quality of your life. Studies show that those who experience a heightened degree of self-focused attention are more likely to suffer from psychological dilemmas and pain. On the other hand, those who give their attention to others and the world around them are happier and more appreciative of their lives. In other words, where you direct your attention may determine the quality of your life.

Learning how to shift your attention is important for your health. In a stressful situation, the way you direct your attention determines the outcome. If you misdirect your attention in a negative direction, your fear and anxiety may increase (stress response). If you direct your attention in a positive way, you may discover a new opportunity to grow (stress resilience).

To shift your attention, begin with your body. Let your body lead your mind, not the other way around. MBX always begins with paying attention to your body and breath. Pay attention to your hands. Progressively move your attention to the arms, head, torso, legs, and then spread your attention to the entire body. *Eventually, your awareness embraces your surroundings*: the floor, ceiling, walls, furniture, music, and all ambient elements. Under ideal conditions, all the ambient elements and you become one. You are aware of yet not consciously thinking. Awareness exists without paying particular attention to it.

A successful experience of MBX practice essentially depends on what kind of attention you give to practicing rather than how long or what movement you perform. Well-guided attention is the key to harvesting the wholistic outcomes of the practice.

In sum, we become what we pay attention to.

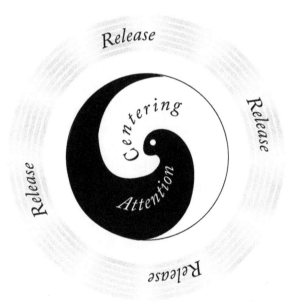

Practice Point: Attention

1. Raise your arms with your hands overlapping. Inhale deeply through your nose.
2. With your hands still above your head, *open your fingers wide* and lower your arms to the side as slowly as you can, maintaining the tension in your hands. Exhale through your mouth. Bring your attention to the sensation of your fingers and arms as you move your arms.
3. Return to a natural standing position with your arms at your side and rest. Feel the residual echoes of the movement in your body.

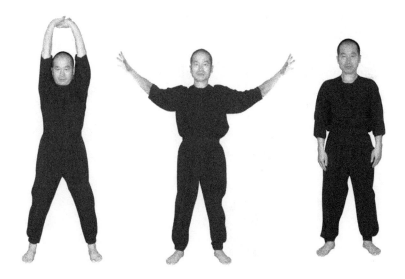

Raise your arms, inhaling deeply. Exhaling, slowly mindfully lower your arms. Stretching your arms and fingers brings your attention intentionally to the body.

CENTERING

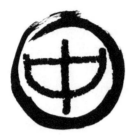

Centering is synonymous with balance. Movement that is well centered or balanced has augmented force and beauty. In this way, physical strength originates in a correctly aligned center. Centering also increases a sense of confidence in the use of the body.

Attention is the first step in discovering our hidden energy. Centering spreads our attention across the body and determines the central point into which the attention flows. The center is located in the lower abdomen area at three fingers' width below and two fingers' depth inward from the navel. This point is known as a reservoir of inner energy and functions as a centering point of stability and physical power. The center is also associated with emotional stability and self-confidence. In martial arts training, for instance, discovering and developing the force of the center is vital for effectiveness in performing physical skills and developing an indomitable spirit. Centering is an active process of building inner strength.

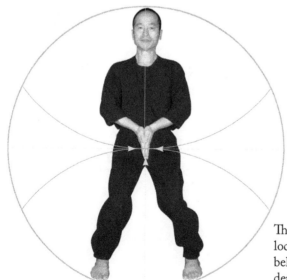

The energy center is located three fingers' width below and two fingers' depth inward of the navel.

Practice Point: Centering

Horse Stance (on the opposite page)

1. Place both feet shoulder width apart. Stand equally on both feet.
2. Slowly bend your legs and lower your body.
3. Put your palms together gently in front of the lower abdomen.
4. Try shifting your balance from foot to foot and up and down to discover where the point of your center is.

Infinity Posture (below)

1. Bend your knees with the heels pointing outward.
2. Place your hands above your head.
3. Take a deep breath in and hold your breath for 3 seconds.
4. Slowly breathe out and lower your body gently by bending your knees.
5. Stop when you feel your lower abdomen becoming tense. That may be the balancing center for your body.
6. For further exploration, to locate your energy center, move your body around with your feet planted.

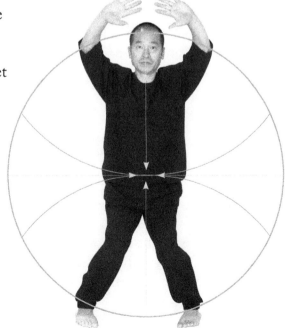

RELEASE

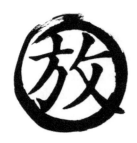 Many illnesses are caused by carrying tension in the body, the result of habitual lifestyle activities. To strengthen the body, the tension must be released.

Release is a transition from 'doing' to 'non-doing' or 'slow-doing'. Doing is directed movement. Non-doing is freedom from directed movement. Slow-doing is a gradual reduction of doing. Doing builds tension in the muscles. Non-doing lets go of the tension in the muscles.

Tension builds up in our body over time. Ironically, when tension is detected, you can use it as a tool to reduce tension by redirecting your attention to the opposite. For example, you feel tightness in the chest. Regardless of the cause, take a few deep breaths and relax for a minute. Then take a really deep breath, expanding your lungs to the maximum and holding for 5 seconds. This builds an even greater amount of tension in your chest. Even better, clench your fist as hard as you can while breathing in. Then let everything go, releasing your breath and fist, not doing anything, just being.

This method of counterbalancing tension using another form of tension is one way to neutralize tension. It channels the tense energy, reminding the region of the body of a previous tension-free condition.

Practice Point: Release

A way to experience non-doing is to stop suddenly in the middle of movement. When you raise your arms (right, photo 1), tension builds. When you stop the movement, there are residual feelings that echo the path of the movement and fill it with a passive sensation of energy. The tension of the movement is replaced with emptiness, which begins to be filled with new sensation, a tension-free feeling.

   Slow-doing is another way to experience tension releasing. After a quick forceful arm raising movement with inhalation (photo 2, below), begin to slowly lower your arms to the sides (photo 3). In that slow movement, dropping your arms like falling petals, there is a sensation of directed release of tension.

   These tension releasing techniques teach the muscles how to unlearn the tension built by a habitual lifestyle and relearn their original status of a tension-free condition.

   Unlearn tension and relearn the tension-free condition of the original body. Mindful movement helps your body return to a balanced tension-free state. This is very important because when understood and practiced properly, you can prevent and cure certain types of nagging pain, even when nothing else seems to work.

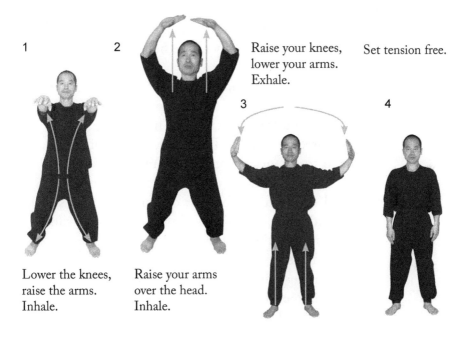

1

2

Raise your knees, lower your arms. Exhale.

Set tension free.

3

4

Lower the knees, raise the arms. Inhale.

Raise your arms over the head. Inhale.

Meridian in Brief

Meridians, *the fourth pillar of energy transformation,* are energy paths that connect to the organs internally and to the limbs and torso externally. On the surface of the meridians, there are accessible vital points that are connected to the brain, organs, and viscera. Most vital points are distributed across the twelve meridian paths and located symmetrically on the right and left sides of the body. These vital points are used to regulate the flow of energy throughout the meridians in Eastern medicine.

There are six meridians on each of the limbs : the first three meridians of the upper limb run from the chest to the hand (Interior or Yin Meridians); the second three meridians of the upper limb run from the hand to the head (Exterior or Yang Meridians); the first three meridians of the lower limb run from the head to the foot (Exterior or Yang Meridians); the second three meridians of the lower limb run from the foot to the abdomen and chest (Interior or Yin Meridians).

The inner energy flows following the order of the twelve meridians (see Summary of MBX-12 table on page 37). When the flow is balanced, the amount of Ki, the inner vital energy, rises.

3
MBX-12

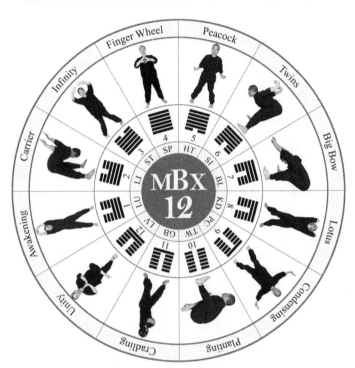

This chapter details step-by-step instruction for the twelve postures that make up the MBX-12 sequence. As you learn and practice the postures, be mindful of the *three principles of practice: attention, centering, and release.* They are, in fact, not separate but one integrative sensation: *the feeling of being one with yourself in the flow.*

Between the instruction for the MBX postures, you will find short readings to help you deepen your knowledge and understanding of the *four pillars of energy transformation: movement, breath, meridians and mindfulness.*

A Brief Overview of MBX-12

MBX-12 consists of twelve mindful movements that activate the twelve meridians in the body. At right is an overview of the order in which the movements should be practiced as well as the associated meridians and anticipated effects. In the pages that follow, the twelve postures are presented in the order they should be learned and practiced.

Initially, practice each posture individually. You can repeat an individual posture up to ten times in one practice session to encourage the development of muscle memory and familiarize your mind and body with the character of the posture. As you feel more comfortable, begin to put the postures together in sequence. It is not necessary to do all twelve postures at first. Take your time and build up to the complete MBX-12 sequence.

As you learn the movements, revisit the descriptions to refine your understanding. Pay special attention to the focus points for each movement, especially as you become more experienced and can give your attention to the finer points of mastery.

The instructional photos that accompany each movement are the ideal postures, however, it may not be possible for you to perfectly imitate every movement. Each of us has a unique body shape and condition. It may be necessary or beneficial to adapt aspects of a movement to fit your body. Experiment with minor adjustments as needed and keep striving to reach the ideal execution of each movement. Don't give up!

Once you are confident that you can perform all twelve movements, practice MBX-12 (movements 1 through 12 in order). Depending on how proficient your practice is, MBX-12 takes three to ten minutes to complete. In the beginning, three minutes is typical. As you advance, the duration of your breath and of holding each posture will lengthen and you will find that MBX-12 takes longer to complete.

You can view a video demonstration of all 12 postures at Youtube (http://www.youtube.com/watch?v=kWE-m6uQOxo) to get a better idea of how to practice them in sequence once you have mastered them individually.

Summary of MBX-12

#	Hexagram	Name	Meridian	Effect
1		Awakening	Lung	Calmness Relaxation
2		Carrier	Large Intestine	Balance Circulation
3		Infinity	Stomach	Energy levels Circulation
4		Finger Wheel	Spleen	Mental balance Self-regulation
5		Peacock	Heart	Equanimity Confidence
6		Twins	Small Intestine	Relax pelvic area Circulation
7		Big Bow	Bladder	Centering Balance
8		Lotus	Kidney	Refreshing Relaxation
9		Condensing	Pericardium	Calmness Perspective
10		Planting	Triple Warmer	Strength Inner power
11		Cradling	Gallbladder	Tranquility Circulation
12		Unity	Liver	Centering Inner energy

The Basics

Stance

There are four basic stances: Natural Stance, Horse Stance, Goat Stance, and Crane Stance. These are explained in detail when they are introduced in the exercises. The illustrations below are simply to familiarize you with stances used in MBX-12 practice.

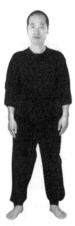

Natural Stance:
Place your feet
one foot apart
and relax.

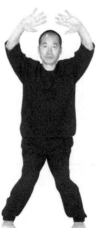

Goat Stance:
From Horse
Stance, rotate the
heels outward 15
to 30 degrees.

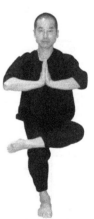

Crane Stance:
Stand on one
leg with knees
bent.

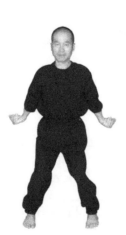

Horse Stance:
The feet are parallel
and knees are slightly
bent.

Postures

There are four types of postures in MBX-12: upright, forward bending, rear arching, and torso twisting.

- **Upright postures** are the most common and easy to practice. Through practicing various upright postures, you can activate meridians located along the limbs and the front of the body.
- **Forward bending postures** activate the meridians located in the rear side of the body and the outside of the arms.
- **Rear arching postures** stretch the meridians located in the front of the body and the inner side of the legs.
- **Torso twisting postures** activate the meridians located along the lateral sides of the body and head.

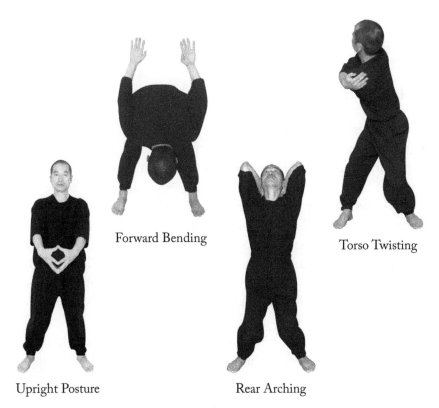

Forward Bending

Torso Twisting

Upright Posture

Rear Arching

Caution

If at any time you feel uncomfortable (for example: dizzy, weak, loss of balance), gently kneel on the floor in the Modified Child Pose or sit down somewhere comfortable. Rest until you completely recover. If the problem persists, stop exercising and consult with your doctor. Further cautions will be indicated as appropriate with individual exercises.

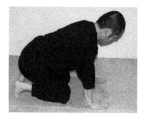

Kneel

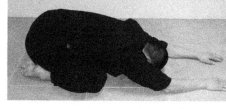

Modified Child Pose

Meridian Basics

Meridians are energy paths connected internally to the organs and externally to the surface of the skin. Each limb has six meridians, three on the inside and three on the outside.

Our inner energy is believed to flow along the meridians in the following order: 1) Lung Meridian, 2) Large Intestine Meridian, 3) Stomach Meridian, 4) Spleen Meridian, 5) Heart Meridian, 6) Small Intestine Meridian, 7) Bladder Meridian, 8) Kidney Meridian, 9) Pericardium Meridian, 10) Triple Warmer Meridian, 11) Gallbladder Meridian, and 12) Liver Meridian.

This 12 meridian cycle repeats every 24 hours. The MBX-12 sequence is designed to stimulate the meridians following this natural cycle.

Repetition and Practice

Repetition is essential to mastering a technique. Through repetitive practice, your muscles and brain remember not only the sequence of movement but also the rhythm and intensity of your performance. In time, practice sets you free from thinking. It helps you flow. Your conscious self merges with the unconscious aspects of self, allowing you to attain a higher realm of practice.

Physically, the sympathetic nervous system become calmer and the activity of the parasympathetic nervous system rises. Your muscles become relaxed, yet your attention becomes sharper. Your mind becomes spontaneously in sync with your body.

Repetition is the key to successful MBX practice. Once you understand how to perform each MBX posture, practice it three to five times and evaluate your performance based on the Self-assessment Criteria (next page). With this self-feedback in mind, practice again three to five times and then reevaluate your performance again until you feel comfortable with the movement. Periodically return to the Self-assessment Criteria as you progress to ensure that your practice retains its physical and mental integrity.

Be mindful that perfection of an exercise may not occur in one or two trials. However, perfection of one single movement, such as raising your arm above your head with a deep inhalation, may be instant.

We are born with natural talent for moving and breathing.

Follow your instincts.

Self-Assessment

Self-assessment is essential to your progress. Here are 4 criteria for evaluating your performance of each posture:

1. Posture

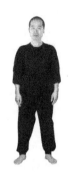

Good posture creates confident feelings about your body. The beginning posture of your practice sets the tone for the subsequent movements. Allow your body to lead your mind. Be restful, yet alert.

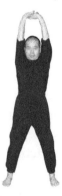
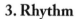

2. Balance

Keep your movement symmetrical by distributing your weight equally on both sides. This enables you to extend your limbs safely through their maximal range of motion while centering the inner energy flow.

3. Rhythm

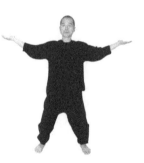

Inhale deeply and exhale slowly. Deep breathing brings you a sense of relaxation and vitality. It generates a rhythmic flow, drawing the mind and the body closer together.

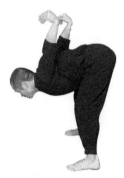

4. Mindfulness

Minimize distractions. Initially, focus your mind only on the present movement. As you advance, the amount of attention you pay to your movement decreases. The separation between the mind and the body vanishes. Only awareness remains.

Connecting the Flow

Each breath has a cyclic life. The air we breathe in enters the nose and the lungs. In the nose, the air mixes with other elements such as nitric oxide, a blood vessel relaxer. In the lungs, oxygen is loaded in hemoglobin and transported to the heart and over five trillion cells.

The cells in our body are the final consumers of everything we take in and the producers of everything we expel. Through this cyclic repetition, we live. When it stops, we die. Repetition is the key for sustaining life forms. Through repetition, the breath fills our cells with new energy from outside which energizes and takes away the rubbish that toxifies. Repetition facilitates the environment in which the mind merges with the body.

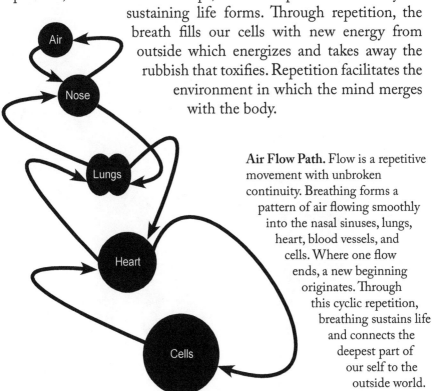

Air Flow Path. Flow is a repetitive movement with unbroken continuity. Breathing forms a pattern of air flowing smoothly into the nasal sinuses, lungs, heart, blood vessels, and cells. Where one flow ends, a new beginning originates. Through this cyclic repetition, breathing sustains life and connects the deepest part of our self to the outside world.

1. Awakening
Lung Meridian

Awakening posture pushes the diaphragm down (1) and stimulates the nerves around the lungs (2-3). This posture also helps you stretch the muscles of the chest and arms, and take in abundant oxygen. During the slow downward movement (3b), extend the thumbs fully to stimulate the lung meridian, which begins under the armpit and ends at the tip of the thumb (diagram on page 46).

1. From a natural stance, inhaling through your nose, raise your arms to the side until your hands are above your head. Do this very slowly and mindfully.

MBX-1

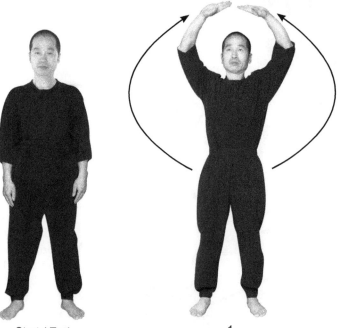

Start / End   1

2. At the top of the extension above your head, overlap your hands together, with the palms facing upward. Inhaling further, as deeply as you can, push your hands upward to maximum extension. At this point, your biceps touch your ears, your spine is erected, and your belly tucked in. Hold this posture for 2-3 seconds.

3. Open your fingers wide (3a). Exhaling slowly, lower your arms to the side (3b). Do this movement very slowly. Feel the inch-by-inch changes along the arms. You may feel an electrical sensation when the arms are lowered halfway. Keep your thumbs extended (the lung meridian passes through here). End in natural stance.

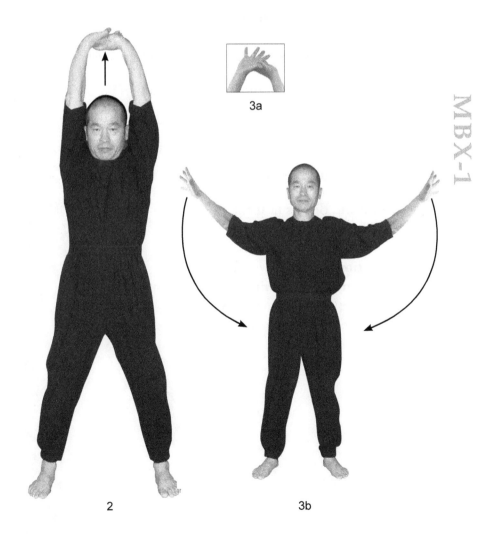

3a

2   3b

Focal Points

- At the top of the stretch, you may hold your breath for 2-3 seconds (optional).
- From this point, lower your arms as slowly as possible (6-10 seconds), bringing your attention to your inner arms. Try to feel the inch-by-inch changes in sensation as your arms descend.
- Extend your thumbs and focus your attention on the Lung Meridian.

Self-assessment Criteria

1. Did you feel a tingling sensation in your arms as your arms descended?
2. Did you control your movement at all time?
3. Do you feel calmer?

MBX-1

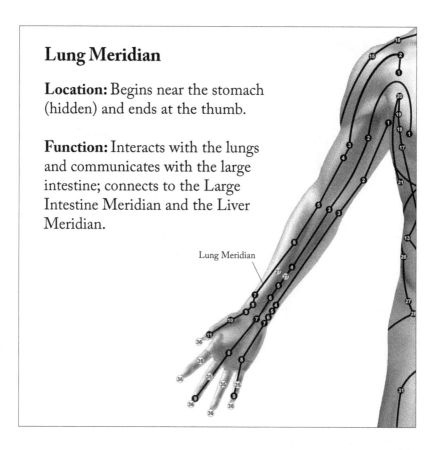

Lung Meridian

Location: Begins near the stomach (hidden) and ends at the thumb.

Function: Interacts with the lungs and communicates with the large intestine; connects to the Large Intestine Meridian and the Liver Meridian.

Lung Meridian

Expected Effects

- Stretching the muscles in the chest
- Stimulation of the Lung Meridians by opening the thumbs
- Activation of parasympathetic nervous system and increased relaxation
- Enhanced self-regulation

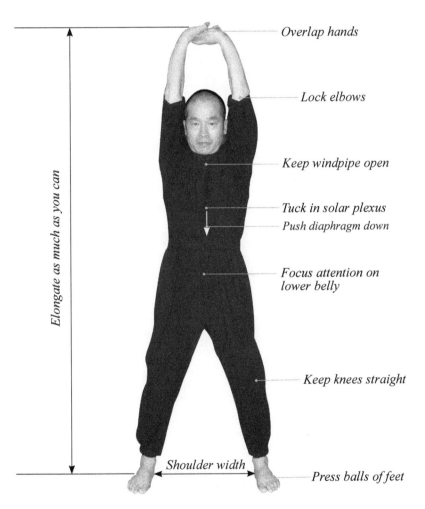

Focal Points of Awakening Posture at full stretch

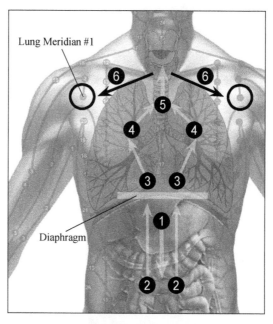

Deep breathing stimulates the pulmonary region, where the Lung Meridian plays a key role. The Lung Meridian originates in the abdomen near the navel (1), goes down through the stomach to the large intestine (2), then turns back upward through the diaphragm (3) to the lung (4). It ascends to the throat (5) and runs transversely to the front surface of the shoulder under the clavicle (6). From the Lung meridian #1 position, the meridian runs along the inner upper arm down to the inner tip of the thumb. Inhalation contracts the diaphragm (downward), and exhalation relaxes it (upward) stimulating the lungs.

Mindful Practice

In Traditional Eastern Medicine, inner energy flows along twelve meridians or energy channels. One complete cycle of the twelve meridians takes 24 hours, with each individual channel's cycle taking approximately two hours.

In keeping with these principles, MBX-12 follows the flow of inner energy along the twelve meridians. When you perform each movement for 15 to 30 seconds, it takes approximately three to six minutes to complete the twelve movements. In this short time, you stimulate all twelve energy channels.

This intense stimulation of the meridians in such a short time period can have a cleansing and vitalizing effect. At times, practice of MBX-12 may push the inner energy into areas that are normally inaccessible due to an energy imbalance or blockage.

Upon completion of one cycle, you may feel relaxed, energized, calm, relieved, fulfilled, strong, balanced, happy, or all of these. However, you may also find that negative or distressing feelings appear. This is normal. When you move mindfully, feeling arises from many sources. Notice the presence of your emotion, but let it be. Don't get caught by positive nor negative emotions. All that is important is the flow. It includes both and excludes neither.

Deep Breathing Methodology

Deep breathing, *the third pillar of energy transformation*, has therapeutic effects on heart rate, blood pressure, and emotional regulation. Studies have shown that deep breathing decreases oxygen consumption, heart rate, and blood pressure, and increases energy levels and parasympathetic activity, leading to a calming effect on the mind and a sense of control of the body.

The basic method used for deep breathing is simple: gently inhale through the nose, briefly hold the breath, and then exhale through the mouth for a duration of twice your inhaling time. When I practice deep breathing, I use the 12-second long, 3-3-6 breath cycle method:

1. Gently breathe in through the nose for 3 seconds.
2. Hold the breath for 3 seconds.
3. Exhale slowly through the mouth for 6 seconds.

When you exhale, form your mouth in the shape of an 'O' and make a soft 'Ho' sound. Slowly contracting the muscles of the abdomen, thorax (chest), and mouth, try to exhale completely.

When you become proficient at deep breathing, one breath takes 15 seconds, meaning you can take four breaths per minute. As you breathe, count the seconds in your mind. Doing so promotes mindfulness and awareness of your practice. In time, you will establish your own natural rhythm and you won't need to count to regulate the duration of each breath.

Note: Always use your common sense when practicing breathing exercises. If you feel uncomfortable, stop and resume after a break.

The Mechanics of Breathing

The mechanics of breathing are relatively simple. When the diaphragm, a dome-shaped muscle under the lungs, moves downward, the pressure in the thoracic cavity and lungs decreases, allowing the air to enter and fill the space. When the diaphragm relaxes, it returns to its original position, facilitating exhalation.

The amount of the air entering and exiting the body depends partially on the range of diaphragm movement. By relaxing and expanding the belly muscles, you can increase the range and breathe more deeply.

The force of the air can be increased or decreased by controlling the speed of breathing and the muscles mobilized for the breath. If you breathe in abruptly and forcefully, the muscles in the rib cage and abdomen expand, increasing the force of the breath. Conversely, if you breathe out slowly and gently, the muscles in the airway, intercostal and abdominal regions relax, eliciting a calming effect on the mind.

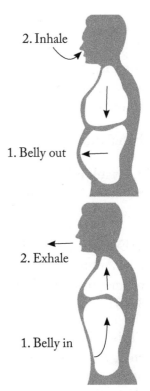

2. Inhale

1. Belly out

2. Exhale

1. Belly in

Breathing Techniques

There are many breathing methods and techniques. Normally we rely on chest breathing, expanding our chest as we inhale. MBX practice, however, focuses primarily on belly breathing.

Belly Breathing Basics

With belly breathing, you expand your lower belly for inhalation and contract the abdominal muscles for exhalation. Here is how belly breathing works:

Inhalation

1. Extend your belly and let the lungs expand.

2. Inhale through your nose. Allow your diaphragm to contract downward as low as possible. This takes 3-5 seconds.

Exhalation

3. At full inhalation, let the extended belly return to the original position slowly.

4. Exhale. Let the diaphragm relax, returning to the normal position. This takes 3-10 seconds.

* It is believed that inner energy circulates in the order of a-j, as shown.

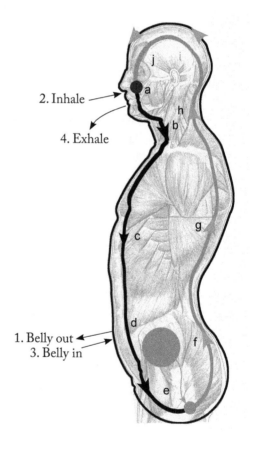

Meridian Breathing

Once you have mastered the belly breathing technique, you may advance to the meridian breathing technique. This method requires imaginative thinking as you conceive and redistribute energy along three energy channels: the Conception and Governing meridians and the Belt channel.

As the belly guides the breath, energy (air) enters the nose and travels down to the belly following the Conception meridian (diagram below, 1), which begins from the perineum and arises along the front of the torso, ending on the chin. The energy gathers and swirls in the belly region encircled by the Belt channel (2). By holding your breath and gently condensing the swirling energy, you can build its strength and push it upward along the Governing meridian (3), which runs along the midline of the back, ascending to the head and descending to the face.

Meridian breathing is a way to distribute energy throughout your body. The Conception meridian connects to all of the Yin meridians (meridians on the inside of the body) and the Governing meridian connects to all of the Yang meridians (meridians on the outside and back of the body). One cycle of meridian breathing connects your inner energy to the external energy of the cosmos.

Meridian breathing is an advanced form of *the third pillar of energy transformation.*

Breath drives inner energy through vertical and horizontal energy channels. 1. Conception meridian (downward flow), 2. Belt channel (swirling flow), 3. Governing meridian (upward flow).

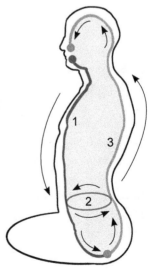

2. *Carrier*

Large Intestine Meridian

Carrier posture activates the Large Intestine Meridian, which extends from exterior upper lines of the index finger to the corner of the nose. Throughout, the index finger leads the movements. While slowly lowering your head and raising your arms, point your index finger to the sky and increase your awareness along the index finger (3). Feel the sensation building along the meridian. When you shift your weight to the rear (4), notice the tension in your hamstrings and the release in the rectum, the end of the large intestine.

1. From natural stance, inhaling, slowly bend your knees and raise your arms upward, with your elbows straight and wrists relaxed in front of you (1).
2. Inhaling further, open your arms to the side, rotating the arms until the palms are facing upward (2).
3. Exhaling, rotate your arms inward until your palms are facing the ground. Gently lower your head and raise your arms vertically behind your back (3).

MBX-2

1   2

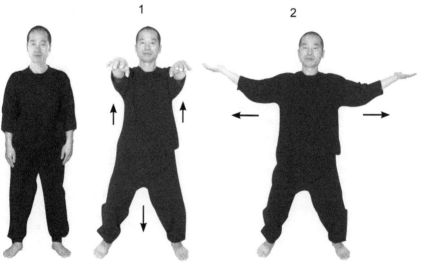

Start / End

4. Inhaling, straighten the knees. Exhaling, shift your weight to your heels and slightly lower your head (4). Breathe normally in this position. Feel the tension in your hamstrings and the release of the pelvic floor. This posture relaxes the muscles of the rectum, the end of the large intestine. Hold this position 3-5 seconds.

5. Inhaling, slowly raise your body, rotating the arms outward until they are extended to your side with the palms facing upward (5). Keep the elbows slightly bent.

6. Exhaling, bring your arms to the front slowly, with the palms facing upward (6).

7. Inhaling, rotate the arms inward quickly (7). Gently lower the arms and exhale. End in natural stance.

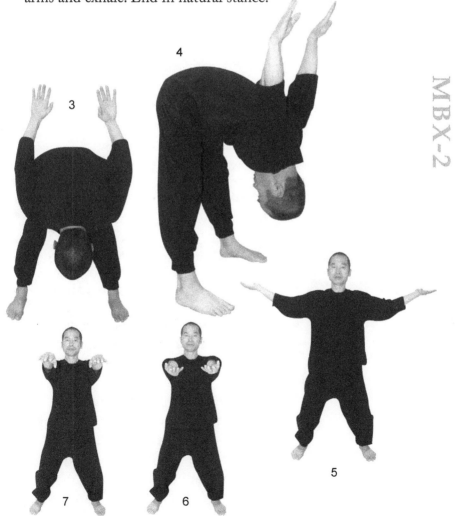

MBX-2

Focal Points

- Generally, move and breathe slowly, except for step 7, which should be done with a quick movement and inhalation.
- At completion of step 2, you may hold your breath for 2-3 seconds (optional).
- In step 3, lower your head and raise your arms as slowly as possible (6-10 seconds). Feel the changing sensation along your inner arms as you move inch-by-inch.
- Be mindful of small changes occurring in the entire body throughout the sequence.

MBX-2

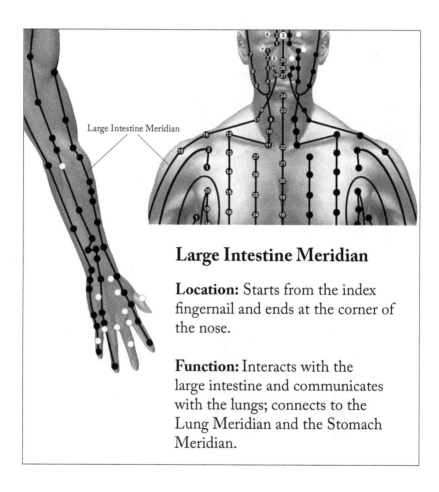

Large Intestine Meridian

Large Intestine Meridian

Location: Starts from the index fingernail and ends at the corner of the nose.

Function: Interacts with the large intestine and communicates with the lungs; connects to the Lung Meridian and the Stomach Meridian.

Self-assessment Criteria

1. Did you notice a feeling of expansion around your chest?
2. Did you feel a stretch in the pelvic muscles?
3. Do you feel the changing sensations along the arms?

Expected Effects

*   Increased sense of balance
*   Feeling of refreshment in the chest area
*   Sense of being unburdened
*   Enhanced blood circulation in the head

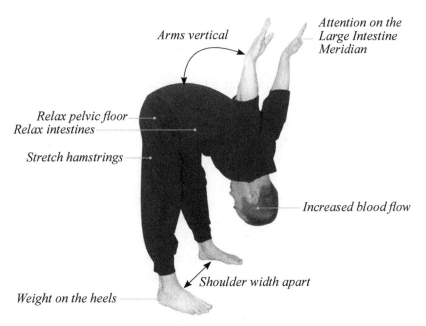

Arms vertical

Attention on the Large Intestine Meridian

Relax pelvic floor
Relax intestines

Stretch hamstrings

Increased blood flow

Shoulder width apart

Weight on the heels

MBX-2

Focal Points of Carrier Posture

Ki: Inner Energy

The first step to discovering your hidden energy is recognizing the presence of a force in you that directs you to do certain things in certain ways. It can be willpower, a string of randomly passing thoughts, spiritual beliefs, feelings, insights, a friend's suggestion, or something that you can't identify. There is something in you that guides you to act or not. It is the force that makes your presence a reality. It awakens your senses to the possibilities of what you are capable of doing, utilizing the force you already have.

An ancient sage wrote that Ki is everywhere. We only need to receive and cultivate it. It is in and around us in all forms and sizes. When we are conscious of the presence of it, we are more likely to be the beneficiary of it. As the old sage said, if you think you know about Tao (the way, for example, of the universe), you don't know about Tao.

The same may be true with Ki. It changes constantly in intensity, magnitude, velocity, and flow. The nature of Ki in the morning and evening is different. The nature of Ki in the spring, summer, fall, and winter fluctuates according to the temperature, the duration of daylight, and the position of the Earth relative to the sun.

During a full moon, your Ki level alters, often in strange ways. The Ki strength of a male may be greater than a female's or vice versa, depending on the personality and mental and physical fitness of the persons. You perhaps have experienced how differently you feel on Monday morning versus Friday morning. Ki alters not only with your fitness levels, environmental and seasonal factors, but also by your attention, intention, and motivation.

Ki is essentially a thing that exists and a living being at the same time. It appears that Ki has the capacity for *self-activation* (the first love affair with the Void), *self-transformation* (in all forms, sizes, and magnitudes), *self-regulation* (with the affinity to both yin and yang energy while being neutral), and *dual-presence* (intangible yet manifesting). Somehow, it contains information which enables it to interact with, influence, and be influenced by other substances. In other words, *you are a participant in the work of this mysterious omnipresent form of energy.*

RECEPTION OF ENERGY

As Ki influences you, your presence also affects the behavior of Ki. More precisely, when you receive Ki, it becomes a meaningful form of energy that lands at its destination. You may not be the intended target of the Ki, but your intention stops and absorbs the Ki. Your intention to consciously be aware of the presence of Ki, such as in the practice of mindful movement, creates a reception station for the Ki. You, as the receiver, become the target of the sender's message (Ki) by your choice.

After all, your reality is a subjective experience. Depending on your energy resources and your intention, the choices you make and the attention you pay will influence the reality you experience.

Your reality is created by your consciousness. For example, you are watching a hummingbird rapidly flapping his wings in midair and meticulously injecting his beak into a hibiscus's tube. When you consciously keep your eyes and ears open, you can see the actions and hear the flapping of the wings. The moment you close your eyes, you are merely partially sensing what the bird is doing.

Only when your eyes are open and you are listening, the visual information of the moving energy of the bird ends up being registered fully (eyes and visual cortex), the sound enters the auditory cortex in the brain, and the information becomes meaningful.

If you don't pay attention, if you don't want it, the information will fly by you. You won't see the amazing feat of the bird. You won't hear anything of the meticulously flying organic thing. The point here is that your subjective reality is determined by your conscious intent. That's why some people may sense Ki and others may not. As the saying goes, beauty truly is in the eye of the beholder. Your choice determines the effects of the Ki.

Similarly, the choices you make about where to live, when to work and rest, and how to live out each day affects the reality you are in and will be in. What this means is that your reality, resulting from your choices, either kills or builds your inner Ki. When it is built, you feel energetic. When it is killed or diminished, you feel tired.

The altered Ki, in turn, can either destroy or motivate your intention. Your intention, for example, to be a great spouse may be compromised due to a lack of or negative Ki, caused by strained relationships or circumstances. This can be changed by replacing your negative Ki with positive Ki, at the same time opting to change your living environment as best as you can. This is possible because *Ki is in constant states of motion, flowing inside and outside of your body.*

INVITING KI IN

The flexibility of Ki is the essence of the life, which characterizes who you are. One can sense the charismatic or optimistic energy when someone like George Clooney walks down the red carpet. Most of us love to be around people with enigmatic energy.

This is not always the case though. Some love the opposite. When the type of Ki is properly matched in relationships, nature nurtures both parties. Although the force of Ki is subtle and intangible as an underlying substance, it is sensible and sometimes obvious. It also varies in form and transforms itself toward balancing the two opposing, yet complementary, forces of yin and yang. It resides simultaneously in both yin and yang, yet Ki itself tends to be neither yin nor yang. It is a neutral base substance, present in all beings.

The day we can know exactly what Ki is and measure it will be the moment we can know how our body communicates and interweaves with the external and internal environment at the cellular and cosmic levels. With your curiosity gently open, Ki may reveal itself for you. With your intention to discover, you may be able to sense the flow of Ki in you and others. Ki flow is a two-way transaction between a giver and a receiver. When you are attentive to Ki, it will find you. When you are receptive, it flows through you. When you interact, you create a new reality within you and become a giver of energy. You become a vital part of this cosmic *Ki dance*.

In summary, from your receptive consciousness, Ki may arise of your own connection with infinitely abundant Ki outside. The Ki from outside (*expressive,* yang Ki) then may merge with the Ki radiating from you (*receptive,* yin Ki) and together find their way through suitable channels in you.

BALANCE OF YIN AND YANG ENERGY

One energy form cannot exist without the other. They attract each other. Where there is yin energy, there is yang energy. The opposite is also true: yang energy repulses yang energy and yin energy repulses yin energy. The traditional *yin-yang diagram* depicts the balanced state of both energy forms.

In reality, however they constantly fluctuate, not only two dimensionally but also in three or four dimensions. For example, in the early morning you may have greater yang energy (active) but in the evening you may have more yin energy (passive).

There are also yang-type or yin-type persons. A yang-type person is characterized by an active and energetic personality whereas a yin-type person is characterized by a calm and unassuming personality.

This typical categorization is not always correct though. The levels of energy can change very rapidly, according to circumstance and the task at hand. An unassuming, generally calm and laid-back, person can turn into an extremely aggressive person. Likewise, a typical yang-type person, always confident and proactive, takes a back seat and becomes indecisive when encountering a stronger yang-type competitor.

Therefore, it is not clear whether one can be a full time yang- or yin-type person, or if the typical categorization is arbitrary. One thing that is clear is that we all have both yin and yang nature; that we can utilize these intrinsic natures by obeying our true self to our best advantage; and that we can transform ourselves to adjust the given nature to meet life's challenges. Clearly, we are born with certain ranges of degree for a yin- or yang-type personality, which may be reflected in our behaviors and thus the course of our life.

There are two other complementary types of energy: innate and acquired. Innate energy is linked with your personality. It has something to do with the way you do things or the way you avoid things. Innate energy is the type of Ki[1] that you are born with (genetic energy, per se). It is the energy that started your heart and lungs.

Acquired energy is the one that you obtain from food and cultivate through activities such as exercise and lifestyle modification. The innate energy is associated with essential levels of vitality and perhaps lifespan. Acquired energy supports the function of innate energy. Your health is achieved when the innate energy is not drained out and the acquired energy levels are sustained at optimum levels.

---

1   The innate Ki is called Jeong in Korean and Chinese. It is one of the three primary energy types of Jeong, Ki, and Shin. Jeong is at the lower energy center in the belly; Ki, the same word as the Ki of essential energy, is at the middle energy center in the chest; and Shin is at the upper energy center in the forehead.

How Does Ki Work?

The questions are then: how does it work and how do we know it works? According to ancient Eastern medicinal philosophers, the human body is equipped with a network of internal energy collectors, called the five organs and six viscera. The five organs include the liver, lungs, spleen, heart, and kidneys. The six viscera are the gallbladder, large intestine, stomach, small intestine, bladder, and triple warmer (an imaginary divider of the torso into upper, middle, and lower sections).

These terms not only refer to the anatomical entities but also to the physiological functions of the body such as circulating blood, receiving and digesting food, absorbing nutrients, and transmitting and removing wastes, following a cyclic natural rhythm.

The ancient philosophers believed that we are all connected. We obtain essential life energy from the earth and from space. When the energy enters the body, it flows through a network of energy channels (meridians) that connect one organ with another. After traveling through cyclic pathways in the body, the energy flows back out to the energy channels of earth and space.

The energy from the earth constitutes the energy of the lower limbs, called yin energy. The energy from space becomes the energy for the upper body, called yang energy. Yin and yang energy meet in the lower abdomen, approximately two inches below the navel, at a one-inch depth into the abdominal cavity. This is called the lower energy center or the *point of conception* (danjeon or dantien).

From this point of conception, Ki flows through twelve meridians, 365 vital points, and two additional energy centers in the middle of the chest and between the eyebrows. When Ki flow becomes weak or blocked, we begin to experience an energy deficit, emotional fragility, and eventually illness. When Ki flows freely through these channels, the organs function properly, stimulating cell growth and reproductivity. Additionally, mental acuity increases and our spirit soars.

The work of Ki reaches between all of the five organs and six viscera, affecting the bodily function, globally and locally. Interwoven with the threads of this energy network, the entire body is impacted by an intangible force.

However, the exact mechanisms of the process have not yet been defined. It is clear that if our energy storage is low, our capacity to actualize our full potential is compromised. This may be what Lao Tzu described as Ki, hidden yet always working, being present everywhere yet found nowhere.

This thousand-year-old myth has fascinated millions of modern health seekers who want to explore a new path along ancient roads. A myth is no longer a myth once you understand it. So you are allowed to get lost in search of Ki. Keep exploring.

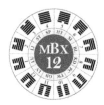

4 PILLARS OF ENERGY TRANSFORMATION

1. Mindfulness: self-generated energy

2. Movement: activity-generated energy

3. Breath: circulation-generated energy

4. Meridians: Ki flow-generated energy

Energy Centers

There are twelve meridians which are linked to the twelve organs and over 365 accupoints. Through these meridians, the body integrates information from the internal and external worlds.

There are seven energy centers and eight energy hubs in the body. The energy centers are where Ki energy is collected and redistributed, whereas the hubs are energy passing stations. Three energy centers are of interest in MBX practice: the lower (in the belly), middle (in the chest), and upper (in the third eye) energy centers.

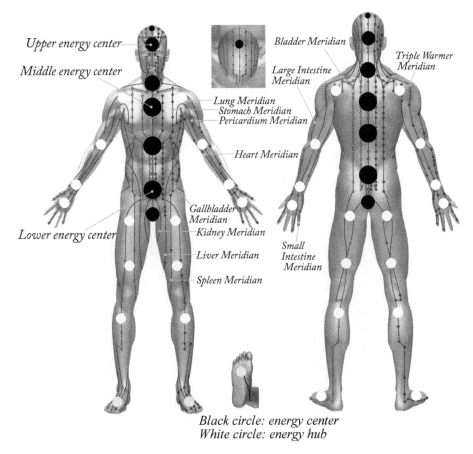

Black circle: energy center
White circle: energy hub

There are over 365 acupressure points along 12 meridians, 7 energy centers in the torso, 4 energy hubs in the upper limbs, and 4 energy hubs in the lower limbs.

3. *Infinity*

Stomach Meridian

Infinity posture increases blood flow to the gut area in two ways: by draining blood from the arms and by pushing blood upward from the legs. Increased blood in the stomach boosts digestion and raises energy levels.

Make sure that you keep your hands at a height that is at least above the head and bend your knees (2). Heels out and toes in. For maximum impact, open your fingers as wide as you can; breathe in through the nose and out through the mouth very slowly.

Be aware of the blood flowing down from the arms to the chest area (the middle energy center) and of the energy surging from the feet to the lower belly (the lower energy center).

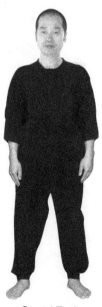

Start / End

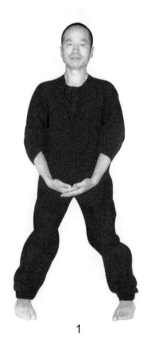

1

1. From natural stance, point your heels outward and bend your knees. Place your open hands in front of your belly with palms facing upward. Exhale.
2. Inhaling, raise your hands above your head with your fingers wide open. Pause for 3 seconds. Exhaling slowly, bend your knees slightly. In the same position, inhale quickly and deeply; then exhale very slowly.
3. Inhaling as deeply as you can, push your hands upward to maximum extension (3a). Slowly exhale while lowering your hands sideways to your hips (3b). Keep your fingers open wide throughout. End in natural stance.

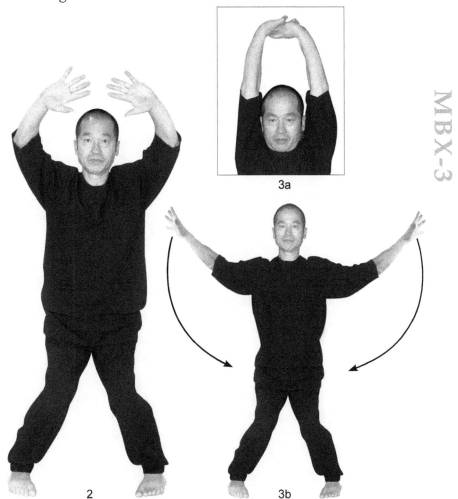

3a

2

3b

Focal Points

- When you are breathing in (2), bring your sensory attention progressively to your fingers, arms, head, chest, stomach, thighs, shins, ankles, and finally your heels.
- Keep your fingers as wide as you can for postures 2 and 3.
- Breathe using the belly muscles at all times: inhale pushing the belly out; exhale by letting the belly return.
- If you are an advanced practitioner, you may stay in posture 2 as long as you wish, depending on your strength. Suggested duration: 15 seconds for beginners, 30 seconds for those who trained for 1 month, 1 minute for those who trained for 2-3 month, 2-5 minutes for those who trained for longer than 3 months.
- For posture 3, stretch your arms in a big circle, taking 5-10 seconds for completion.

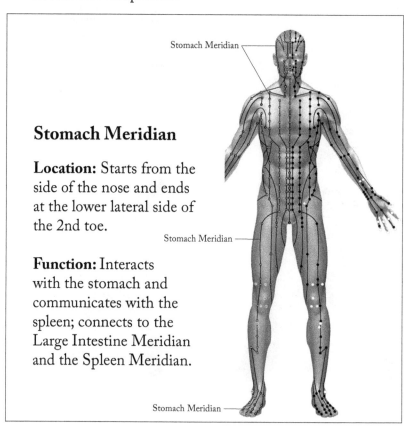

Stomach Meridian

Stomach Meridian

Stomach Meridian

Stomach Meridian

Location: Starts from the side of the nose and ends at the lower lateral side of the 2nd toe.

Function: Interacts with the stomach and communicates with the spleen; connects to the Large Intestine Meridian and the Spleen Meridian.

MBX-3

Self-assessment Criteria

1. Did you feel a tingling sensation in the arms?
2. Did you feel the surging energy from the lower limbs?
3. Do you feel increased strength?

Expected Effects

- Increased sense of balance and strength
- Enhanced mental and physical calmness
- Sense of self-regulation

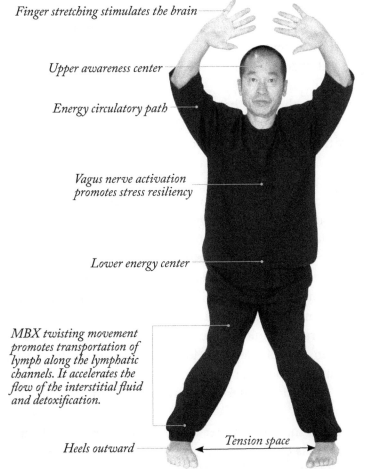

Finger stretching stimulates the brain

Upper awareness center

Energy circulatory path

Vagus nerve activation
promotes stress resiliency

Lower energy center

MBX twisting movement
promotes transportation of
lymph along the lymphatic
channels. It accelerates the
flow of the interstitial fluid
and detoxification.

Heels outward

Tension space

Integrative systemic effects of the Infinity Posture

MBX-3

Twisting the Limbs

Twisting of the limbs and torso is an important part of MBX practice. It augments the beneficial effects of contracting the muscles via coiling and uncoiling actions.

Why is this important?

In our body, the areas between our organs, muscles, bones and other structures, are known as interstitial space. The interstitial areas are filled with fluid, which is managed by the lymphatic system, a series of accessory channels and nodes. When interstitial fluid enters the lymphatic channels, the fluid forms lymph, which flows though one-way channels that flow toward the heart. The primary function of the lymphatic system is to regulate the pressure and volume of interstitial fluid as well as the protein concentration in the fluid.

Normally the interstitial pressure is negative, encouraging fluid to flow into the lymphatic channels. This negative balance promotes detoxification of the body by facilitating a steady outflow of toxins from the surrounding organs, muscles and other tissues.

If the interstitial fluid pressure becomes positive, fluid fills the spaces between tissues causing edema, which we see in the form of swelling in our joints or limbs. Instead of draining from the body, toxins and other wastes accumulate in the interstitial fluid or adjacent tissue.

As you can imagine, proper drainage of excess fluid from the interstitial space is crucial. An efficiently working lymphatic system not only prevents unhealthy swelling, it is also one of our body's most powerful natural healing tools, targeting and removing harmful bacteria, viruses and toxins as well as delivering nutrients to the cells. While the lymphatic channels work quite well on their own, we can accelerate mobilization of lymph in the lymphatic channels by intrinsic and extrinsic compressions of the lymphatic vessels and the contractions of skeletal muscles.

MBX flow exercise promotes transportation of lymph along the lymphatic channels. The unique twisting movements in particular augment the benefits of muscle contractions. The mechanical coiling and uncoiling action of the limbs and torso accelerate the flow of the interstitial fluid and the detoxification process.

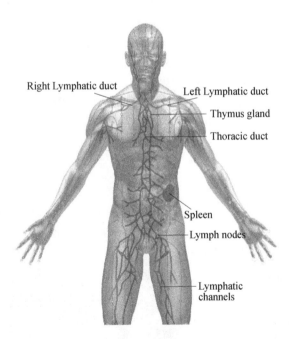

The Lymphatic System. The lymphatic fluid flows through network of channels, vessels and nodes in the torso and limbs.

4. Finger Wheel
Spleen Meridian

Finger Wheel stimulates the fingers, toes, thighs, and torso along the Spleen Meridian, which begins from the lower medial side of the big toenail and ends under the armpit.

Imagine that you are holding a ball (with your fingers wrapped around it, finger tips touching) in front of the belly (1); inhaling, move the ball up to the chest (the middle energy center) (2); exhaling, lift your heels and throw the ball dynamically toward the front (3); and finally bring the ball down to a spot in front of the belly (the lower energy center) (4).

Your toes are facing outward diagonally, so that upon lifting the heels the energy surges upward (3) from the thumb toes, along the inner legs, to the spleen and kidneys.

The spleen is stimulated when, exhaling (3-4), you tuck the belly inward as much as possible. Practicing slowly helps you develop a sense of connectedness among the fingers and toes, and the chest and belly. This exercise elicits a calming effect on the brain by synchronizing the activities of the left and

MBX-4

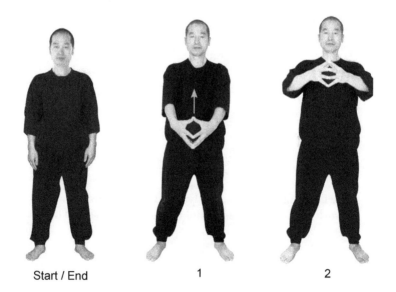

Start / End   1   2

right hemispheres. Finger Wheel also activates the proprioceptors (sensors that detect changes in muscle length and tension) in the limbs increasing the sense of balance.

1. From natural stance with your toes pointed slightly outward, place your hands in front of the lower abdomen with your fingertips pressing against each other (1).
2. Inhaling quickly by pushing the belly out, raise your hands to chest level with elbows bent (2).
3. Exhaling, lift your heels briskly off the floor and roll your hands forward (3) in a circular motion ending in posture 4. For exhalation, initially breathe out sharply, then slow down commensurate to the speed of the fall of the hands. As the imaginary energy ball in your hands begins to fall, lower it as slowly as possible, like a feather falling.

Repeat 3-5 times.

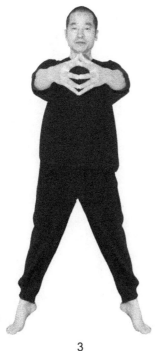

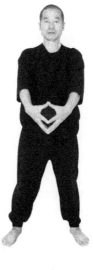

3   4

Focal Points

- The theme of Finger Wheel is rhythmic circular movement.
- You may alter the intensity of the fingertip press and the phase of the rolling movement. For example, raise your hands quickly, pressing the fingertips together hard. Follow with a slow downward movement, gently pressing your fingertips together. (Or vice versa.)
- When you slowly lower your heels, imagine being as light as falling snowflakes landing on the ground.

Four Point Tension: When you lift your heels, tension occurs simultaneously at four points: toes, belly, solar plexus, and fingertips. Synchronize this tension with your inhalation.

The spleen, an organ in the upper left side of the abdomen, is the size of your fist and about four inches long. The spleen filters blood and plays key roles in the function of the immune system including storing white blood cells and assisting the fight against invading bacteria.

MBX-4

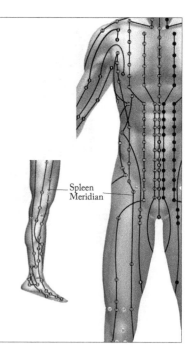

Spleen Meridian

Location: Starts from the lower medial side of the big toenail and ends under the armpit.

Function: Interacts with the spleen and communicates with the stomach; connects to the Stomach Meridian and the Heart Meridian.

Spleen
Meridian

Self-assessment Criteria

1. Did you feel the upward surging energy in your legs upon lifting the heels?
2. Did you squeeze the belly inward during exhalation?
3. Did you feel that your toes, legs, fingers, and torso were moving in synchronization? If not, slow down a bit.

Expected Effects

- Stimulation of the nerves in the toes and fingers
- Increased sense of balance
- Increased calmness

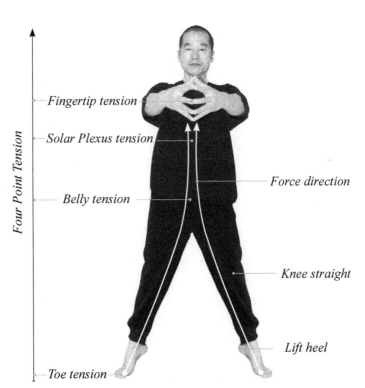

Focal Points of Finger Wheel

Selective Senses

Our brains are bombarded with millions of bits of sensory information per second. Many sensory triggers demand your attention, but your resources are limited. You choose to pay attention to what is useful and ignore the useless sensory noise that makes up most of the incoming data.

In this way, sensory inputs make you aware of your priorities. When you have specific wants or goals, your brain selects specific information to act on. You become an efficient decision maker. Consequently, you can use this natural tendency of your brain to filter and organize information as a problem solving strategy.

Try it: take time to mindfully plant the seed of a question in your mind. This type of active questioning activates the sensory screening area of your brain, giving it a specific "mission" to complete. Out of those millions bits of sensory information you receive, you are now selectively looking for the cues that may provide you with answers to your question.

Even after you stop actively thinking about that question, your brain continues to sort through incoming data and search existing data, looking for answers. In the same way that you continue to experience positive physical effects for 72 hours after exercising, once you initiate mindful practice, your brain continues to benefit from that mindful state for many hours afterward.

Don't be surprised if the answer to your question appears when you least expect it—when you are showering or walking the dog or about to fall asleep. These aha! moments are one of the joyful side benefits of practicing mindfulness.

Circadian Impacts

In Eastern Medicine, our internal energy flow completes one cycle in 24 hours. Beginning from the Lung meridian between three and five AM, our inner energy follows a specific route through the body, with each meridian occupying a two-hour period of the cycle. If you find this hard to understand, imagine it this way: the energy "visits" each of the twelve meridians for a two-hour period, delivering vital information and putting the meridian's "house" in order.

This 24-hour cycle is much like our body's circadian rhythm, a 24-hour cycle that is primarily influenced by the cycle of light and darkness in our environment. As part of our circadian cycle, the body naturally adopts certain internal biorhythms that regulate our sleep-wake cycles, hormonal secretion, mood, and metabolism in anticipation of rhythmic changes in our environment.

Light is the primary factor influencing circadian rhythms, acting like a switch that regulates the body's internal clocks. Scientists believe that the suprachiasmatic nucleus (SCN), a cluster of nerve cells in the brain, may be the master internal clock. Recently, additional internal clocks, called *peripheral oscillators*, have been identified in the organs such as the esophagus, lungs, liver, pancreas, spleen, thymus, and even in the skin.

Practicing the MBX-12 sequence can help balance both the meridian cycle and the circadian cycle. MBX-12 stimulates the meridians in the same order that our natural energy cycle follows, promoting organ and system health, improving sleep habits, boosting mood, and reducing the discrepancy between our internal and external environments.

Fluidity of Movement

By nature, the human body is created to be physical. It is designed to move around for hunting, gathering and exploring the world. Because of the body's highly adaptive nature and physical mobility, we have survived for millions of years.

In addition to survival, movement plays a critical role in making us aware of who we are as human beings. Movement fosters creativity in critical thinking and problem solving. We express our thoughts and feelings through movement. We think, act, learn, and discover through movement or play.

In creative movement, our thoughts flow. This experience of fluid thinking leads to more fluid movement. Fluid movement in turn allows us to be flexible in thinking, enhancing our mood, creativity, and motivation.

Fluidity of movement energizes our life force.

When fluidity of movement is lost, the body easily loses its physical balance and often its functional capacity. Once broken, we become susceptible to injury, loss of self-confidence, and other maladies.

By moving, we build the essential element of life: our sense of self. We can control our movement at will, and in turn we can control how we perceive ourselves.

Movement is a vehicle that brings all of our senses together, enabling us to sense self as a whole.

Calming the Nerves

The torso is home to the widely webbed vagus nerve, which connects the brain with the organs and influences our emotion, appetite, and energy level. When you raise your arms above your head, you naturally breathe in, expanding your torso and stretching the muscles surrounding the organs. This movement stimulates the vagus nerve, naturally activating the calming properties of the parasympathetic nervous system and deactivating the arousal properties of the sympathetic nervous system.

Activation of the parasympathetic nervous system, which is responsible for the body's "rest and digest" functions, shifts the body's physiologic condition from arousal mode to relaxation mode. This physiologic shift is associated with a reduction in heart rate and blood pressure and an increase in calmness and emotional self-regulation. Studies have also shown that stimulation of the vagus nerve reduces tissue swelling, enhances executive functions of the brain, slows cell activity, balances the nervous system, and harmonizes the activities of the major organs such as the heart, lungs, and kidneys.

Because it is effective at triggering the body's natural relaxation response, practice of MBX-12 can be a pathway to de-escalating physical arousal such as stress or anxiety. When you find your heart rate is rising or your breathing is becoming irregular due to unwanted emotional arousal, take a few moments to breathe deeply while practicing Awakening (MBX-1) or Infinity (MBX-3) posture.

5. *Peacock*

Heart Meridian

Peacock posture induces tranquility in the heart and builds your inner strength. By activating the Heart Meridian, which begins from the heart and ends at the inner tip of the little finger, practice of Peacock posture can slow the heart rate and lower blood pressure.

This exercise begins from a calm stable stance, with both hands overlapped in front of the lower energy center (1), which generates a sense of composure. A deep inhalation (2-3) pushes the diaphragm down, producing a feeling of strength and restful alertness. A long exhalation, with slow stretching of the meridian from the heart to the little finger (4-5), expands your chest completely.

Make your hands like two bird beaks and bend them toward your wrists as tightly as you can. When you lower them very slowly, from the top of your shoulders to the sides of the hips, you will feel the intensity of your inner energy built up in the body.

MBX-5

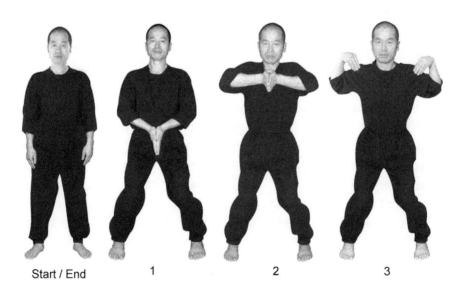

Start / End   1   2   3

1. From natural stance, place your heels outward and bend your knees. Overlap your palms in front of the lower abdomen with the fingers pointing downward. Exhale.
2. Inhaling, bring your hands up to chest level with both palms pressing against each other.
3. Inhaling further, toss both hands to the top edges of the shoulders. At this time, keep your hands like bird beaks. Press the thumb, index, and middle finger against each other, pointing at your biceps.
4. Exhaling, very slowly lower your elbows toward the rib cage, then move your bent hands along the arms. Breathe out through your mouth (with "Hah" sound). Sink your shoulders.
5. When you've completed lowering your hands, return to natural stance.

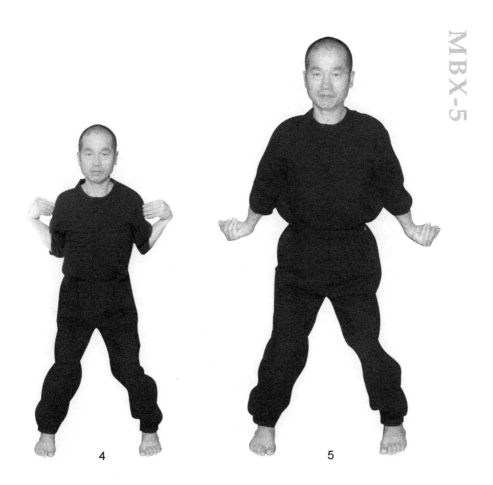

4   5

MBX-5

Focal Points

- Pay special attention to your hands (bend them firmly), elbows (keep them close to the torso), and shoulders (sink, lower, relax but firmly control).
- Exhale slowly (6-10 seconds) with force through your mouth.
- Feel the tension in the entire torso and arms.
- Be aware of the sensation of release after the tension is dissipated.

MBX-5

Heart Meridian

Location: Starts from the heart and ends at the lower medial corner of the small fingernail.

Function: Interacts with the heart and communicates with the small intestine; connects to the Spleen Meridian and the Small Intestine Meridian.

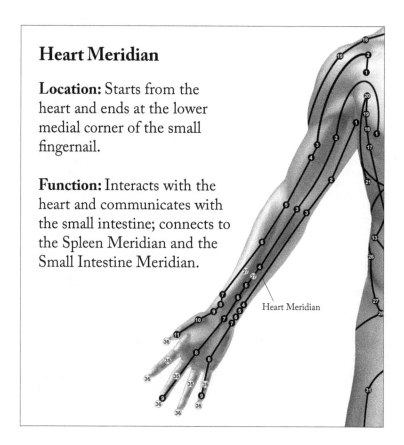

Heart Meridian

Self-assessment Criteria

- Did you feel extraordinary tension and strength in your torso and arms?
- Did you feel calmness when you expanded the chest?
- Did you feel increased relaxation afterward?

Expected Effects

- Increased sense of balance and strength
- Enhanced mental and physical calmness
- Enhanced restful alertness
- Sense of relief

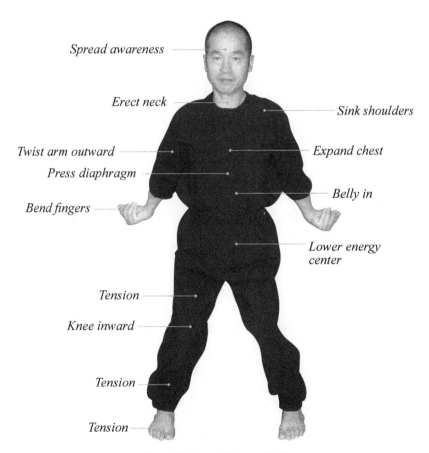

Spread awareness

Erect neck

Sink shoulders

Twist arm outward

Expand chest

Press diaphragm

Belly in

Bend fingers

Lower energy center

Tension

Knee inward

Tension

Tension

Focal Points of Peacock Posture

Impact on Circulation

Movement affects the circulatory system in immediate and lasting ways. In the short term, it causes blood to move differently than when we are at rest. For example, raising the arms above the head causes blood to flow downward into the torso, increasing the blood volume in the organs. Other postures direct blood flow to the head (bending forward), limbs (lowering arms below the heart), and torso (squatting and contracting leg muscles).

Movement and changes in posture also change the blood dynamics in the body. For instance, when the parasympathetic nervous system is activated by stimulating the vagus nerve, vasodilation occurs. As a result, the size of the blood vessels increases and blood pressure decreases.

When you combine the effects of mindful movement with deep breathing, the positive impact becomes even greater. Deep breathing enhances the mixture of nitric oxide and inhaled gases in the nasal cavity, resulting in increased blood vessel flexibility and a greater supply of blood to the heart, lungs and brain.

Relaxed, flexible blood vessels carry more blood and oxygen to the tissues. Better circulation transports more nutrients, gases, and wastes to and from cells, helps fight disease, and encourages the body's natural tendency to seek an internal balance, fostering an optimal inner environment.

This combination of mindful movement and deep breathing has the synergic effect of improving circulation, by generating whole body relaxation, a hallmark of MBX.

Blood Follows Ki

In traditional Eastern Medicine, there is a belief that blood flow follows Ki. Where there is strong Ki, blood flows with force. Where Ki is low, blood flows weakly. In individuals with optimal Ki flow (those who are healthy, confident, mentally acute), there is a balance in circulating Ki which allows blood to flow into tissues evenly throughout the body with sufficient nutrients and oxygen.

An increase in Ki level is also believed to strengthen the immune system. We might find evidence to support this belief in modern science. Meditation or yoga practice is associated with increases in hormones and immune system components (beta-endorphin, serotonin, dopamine, and T-cell secretion) and reduction in anxiety and stress response. This may explain why people who practice mindful movement or meditation are not only healthier but feel better. Eastern medicine practitioners would say that strong Ki contributes to these outcomes.

How can you sense the strength of your Ki flow? Remember that blood follows Ki. Try a simple exercise: slowly raise your arms, place your fists behind your head (Lotus posture, page 99), and gently tilt your head back, rasing your elbows. Hold that position for ten seconds. Notice the gradually changing sensations. Let your mind go along with the flow.

If you don't feel it, don't worry. You will discover it as you become more experienced with mindfulness practice. Ki is hidden, but by practicing MBX you will experience it.

6. Twins

Small Intestine Meridian

Twins posture stimulates the Small Intestine Meridian, which connects the small intestines with the vital energy channels in the side of the skull and the back of arms. This posture facilitates the inner environment for intestinal relaxation and improves blood circulation in the stomach and brain (3). These effects improve digestion, nutritional absorption, and cognitive function.

Once you've bent the torso, straighten your legs and shift your weight forward (4). You will experience increased pressure under the bottoms of the first toes which releases tension in the pelvic floor. Alleviation of tension in the pelvic floor, in turn, helps the intestine relax. You may stay in this posture (4) as long as you want, but be cautious of flooding the head with blood. If you feel uncomfortable or light-headed, gently kneel and go to modified child pose.

MBX-6

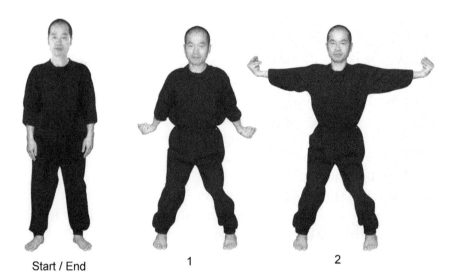

Start / End   1   2

1. From natural stance, place your heels outward and bend your knees. This is the ending position of Peacock posture (MBX-5). Exhale.
2. Inhaling, raise your arms to shoulder height on your sides.
3. Exhaling, slowly bend your body forward and raise your arms backward while rotating your arms inward.
4. Inhaling, straighten your legs. Exhaling, shift your weight to your toes, raising your arms backward vertically and lowering your head as much as you can while looking at the ground. Hold for 5-10 seconds while breathing normally. *
5. Slowly raise your body and return to natural stance.

   If you become dizzy, slowly kneel and go to modified child pose (kneeling with upper body bent forward, arms relaxed and forehead gently resting on the floor).

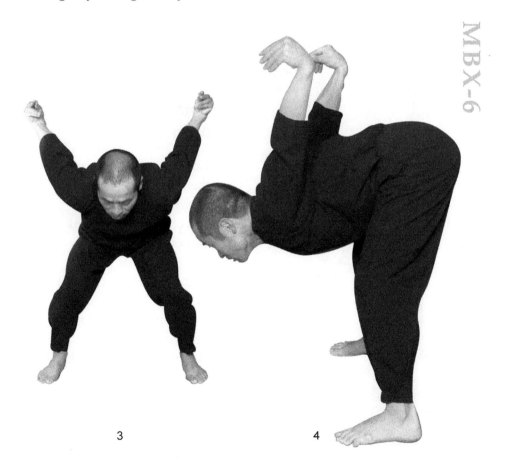

3   4

Focal Points

- Move and breathe slowly.
- Positions 3 and 4 should take 6-15 seconds.
- When you raise your arms, feel the gradually changing sensation along your arms.
- When you lower your head, you will feel blood flooding into your head, so go slowly.
- In position 4, keep your torso down but look up so that you can feel the stretch in your facial muscles. If looking up is uncomfortable for your neck, keep your head at a comfortable angle, looking at the floor.

MBX-6

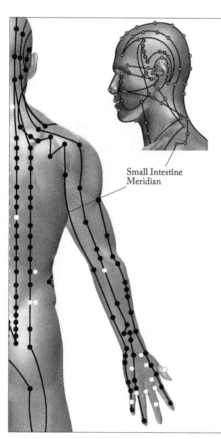

Small Intestine
Meridian

Small Intestine Meridian

Location: Starts from the lateral side of the tip of the small fingernail and ends at the medial corner of the eye.

Function: Interacts with the small intestine and communicates with the heart; connects to the Heart Meridian and the Bladder Meridian.

Self-assessment Criteria

1. Did you feel altering sensations along the arms as you raised your arms backward?
2. Did you feel the pressure under the first toes?
3. Did you experience alleviated tension in the pelvic floor and subsequent relaxation in the abdomen?

Expected Effects

- Increased sense of balance
- Enhanced mental and physical calmness
- Tension relief in the intestines

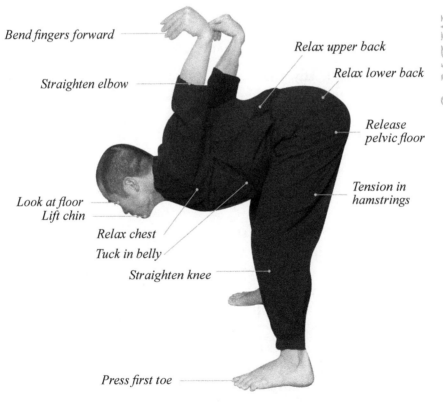

Bend fingers forward

Straighten elbow

Relax upper back

Relax lower back

Release pelvic floor

Look at floor
Lift chin

Relax chest

Tuck in belly

Straighten knee

Tension in hamstrings

Press first toe

MBX-6

Focal Points of Twins

Stress Resilience

Stress resilience is the capacity to rebound from the negative impacts of stress or being immune to typical stressors. There are three steps we can take to attain stress resilience: 1) reduce the stress response, 2) practice mindfulness, and 3) adopt lifestyle changes.

STEP ONE: REDUCE STRESS RESPONSE

Directly or indirectly, you have to eliminate or reduce the size of the stressors and you should do it immediately. You might be able to reduce or eliminate stress quickly by acting on a problem or engaging in vigorous activity. However, often there is nothing we can do about an acute stressor.

STEP TWO: PRACTICE MINDFULNESS

When you cannot remove the stressors, practicing mindful movement with deep breathing is a way to elicit positive physiologic responses by activating the parasympathetic nervous system. MBX-12 stimulates the vagus nerve, the longest cranial nerve connecting the brain and organs, which shifts the body's physiologic response from sympathetic (arousal) to parasympathetic (relaxation). Stimulation of the vagus nerve is also associated with improved emotional self-regulation, executive functions in the brain, and neuroendocrine functions, which positively contribute to mental health and stress resilience.

STEP THREE: CHANGE YOUR LIFESTYLE

Chronic stress is often related to a mental, physical or situational condition that we are unable to adjust to. To cope with it, we need to change the way we respond and to have outlets to buffer its negative impacts. In other words, we need to create a lifestyle change.

An invaluable step in changing your lifestyle is setting a goal to lead a stress-resilient life. With a specific goal in mind, you can reverse your situation from passive to proactive. Your horizon widens. As you gain more options, the buffer zone in your mind grows.

Then, you can monitor stressors as you might watch cars passing under a highway bridge. You can choose to observe which stressor is yours. You are no longer simply reacting but responding with a positive goal of coping with the stressor.

Specifically, how can you set this goal of becoming stress-resilient in motion? By identifying problems through observation and then setting the direction of your effort to solve the problems. You do not need to solve the problem immediately. Simply setting yourself in motion along the right path is enough at the start. It appears to be a small step, especially if the problem is large, but ultimately it is *a game changer*. Now you are paying close attention to problematic stressors, tackling them before they overwhelm you. Revolution quietly starts within.

Your interactions with your body impact stress resilience. Activities to increase your interactions within you include, but are not limited to, martial arts, taichi, yoga, meditation, jogging, swimming, rock climbing, talking, movie watching, guitar playing, reading, lovemaking, and traveling.

Writing, in the form of journaling or blogging, is also an excellent way to reduce your stress. More importantly, it helps you understand who you are and why you are the way you are, liberating yourself from a "have-to-be" perfectionist to an "I-am-what-I-am-and-I-like-it" pragmatist.

Synergistically, you will sleep better, eat better, and feel better about yourself. You will be less tired, more active, and more productive. Realistically, changing your lifestyle is the best way to take care of yourself.

7. Big Bow
Bladder Meridian

Big Bow posture stretches the entire back: the bottom of the foot, calf, thigh, lower back, and upper back. This exercise activates the Bladder Meridian, which begins as two channels originating from the inner corner of the eyes, rises to the top of the skull, descends to the neck, and splits into four channels in the back, merging into two channels again in the rear thigh, then merging again into one channel in the upper calf, and ending at the lateral side of the tip of the little toe.

The Bladder Meridian communicates with the brain, and connects the kidney and urinary bladder. Big Bow posture stimulates these organs and induces positive effects such as improved circulation and relaxation as well as reduced blood pressure and anxiety.

You should practice this posture very slowly to prevent dizziness and loss of balance. The key movement is Tilting Stretch (3b) in which you stretch your arms forward and the

MBX-7

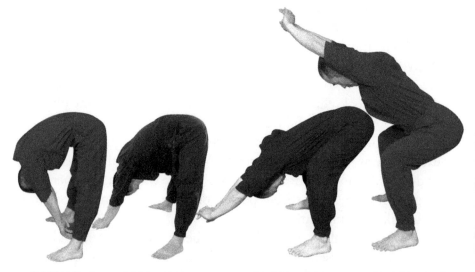

5 (side view)   4 (side view)   3b (side view)   3a (side view)

buttocks backward as far as you can while exhaling. (You may place your hands on the floor for better anchoring.) Then lift your hip slightly to release the tension in the pelvic floor and the lower back while keeping your hands close to the floor (4).

1. From natural stance, inhaling, stretch your arms as high as you can with one hand overlapping the other and the palms facing upward.
2. Exhaling, slowly lower your stance.
3. Inhaling, slowly bend your body forward and reach your hands out to the front until your hands reach the floor (3a-3b).
4. Exhaling, lift your hip slightly and stretch your arms further forward (or place your hands on the floor). Feel the release in the lower back.
5. Inhaling, very slowly arch your back and bring your body up to natural stance.

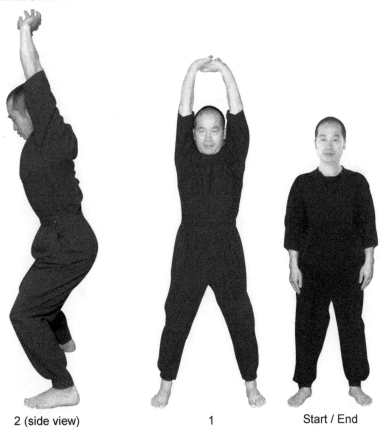

2 (side view)   1   Start / End

Focal Points

- If you have a history of back pain or injury, consult with your doctor first.
- *You may modify this posture by placing your hands on a table or other sturdy surface at hip height* to prevent strain in the back.
- Before bending, you should balance your body first by lowering your stance.
- Keep your hands together when bending so that you have firm control of your torso.
- As you reach out, adjust your posture or lower your stance to gain the best control of your body.

MBX-7

Bladder Meridian

Location: Starts from the corner of the eye, rises to the top of the skull, descends to the back, and ends at the lower lateral corner of the small toenail.

Function: Interacts with the urinary bladder and communicates with the kidney; connects to the Small Intestine Meridian and the Kidney Meridian.

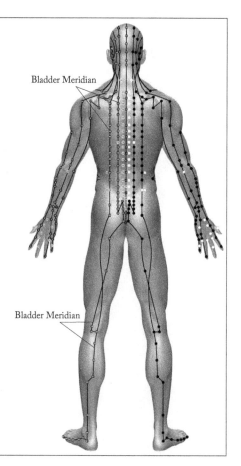

Bladder Meridian

Bladder Meridian

Self-assessment Criteria

1. Did you experience a good sense of stretching in your back?
2. Did you control your movement at all times?
3. Are you experiencing less tension in your back afterward?

Expected Effects

- Increased sense of strength
- Alleviation of tension in the body
- Enhanced sense of wholeness

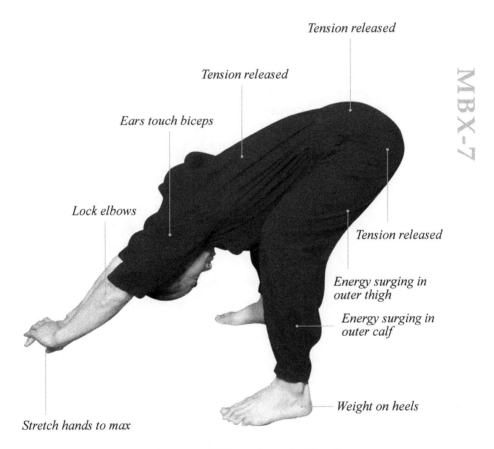

Tension released

Tension released

Ears touch biceps

Lock elbows

Tension released

Energy surging in outer thigh

Energy surging in outer calf

Weight on heels

Stretch hands to max

Focal Points of Tilting Stretch of Big Bow

Proprioception

After the senses of sight, smell, hearing, taste, and touch, proprioception is regarded as the sixth sense. Derived from the Latin word meaning 'sense of self', proprioception is a position-movement sensation based on information about the relative position of the parts of our body in space. This sense of position is initiated by proprioceptors located in the joints and muscles, which transmit information about joint angle, muscle length, and muscle tension to the brain.

In addition to information received from the limbs, proprioception is influenced by sensory neurons in the inner ear, which contributes to our sense of motion and orientation in space. Finally, the cerebellum, a small area at the rear of the brain, plays a key role in body control and balance. Regardless of which pathway the body uses to transmit proprioceptive signals, they are processed in the cerebellum.

Without proprioception, we would be physically confused and clumsy. It would be difficult to sense the position of our arms or legs in relation to our body and we would struggle to adjust how much strength to use when picking up objects.

As we age, we often suffer from a decreased sense of proprioception, which contributes to increased loss of balance and falling. We can counter this natural decline by purposely stimulating our proprioceptive receptors. Standing on one leg (Infinity posture) or tilting multiple parts of the body in one position (Big Bow and Lotus postures) is a simple, effective way to increase proprioceptive feedback. Sound proprioceptive feedback balances your senses and helps integrate your physical self-perception.

Change Your Mood

Breathing not only helps us sustain life but also calms us under stress and marshals our power when we feel weak. Think about how your breathing reflects your current physical and mental status. When you are calm, you take even, regular breaths. Similarly, long deep breaths manifest a relaxed or surrendered status.

As your emotional condition changes, your breathing pattern changes. When you are upset or anxious, your breathing becomes irregular, marked by short rapid breaths. Why? The activation of the fight or flight response. Just as your breathing becomes more rapid during exercise, it also speeds up as anxiety rises, increasing the oxygen in your cells in preparation for fighting or fleeing.

In the same way that your mood affects your breathing, your breathing can impact your mood. When you are anxious, take a few deep breaths and soon you feel less anxious. When you feel down, take a few forceful breaths in and out, and you'll feel uplifted. When you change your breathing pattern, your emotional condition changes.

Deep breathing promotes calmness, improves awareness, and increases energy levels. Just think of a time when you were upset and someone counseled you to "take a deep breath" or "just breathe." Intentionally slowing your breathing sends a signal to your brain and body: relax. Conversely, short and fast breathing is a good way to increase alertness and vigor by increasing activity at the cellular level. Often a conscious change in your breathing pattern is the first step to redirecting negative energy into positive energy.

8. Lotus

Kidney Meridian

Lotus posture stimulates the bottom-most energy center, the feet, and compresses the kidneys. Under the bottom of the feet is the gate for energy from mother earth to enter our body. It is a root energy that surges into the body through the Kidney Meridian, resonating with nourishing life force. Our health and happiness in life is enriched by this motherly nourishment.

Starting from the bottom of the foot, innervating through the inner leg toward the groin and up the front of the pelvis, and ending at the upper central region of the chest, the Kidney Meridian is known as the most influential and mythical energy channel for stamina and reproductive function in humans.

Lotus posture consists of two simple movements: natural stance and Head Rest (2). Each repetition takes only 10 seconds.

MBX-8

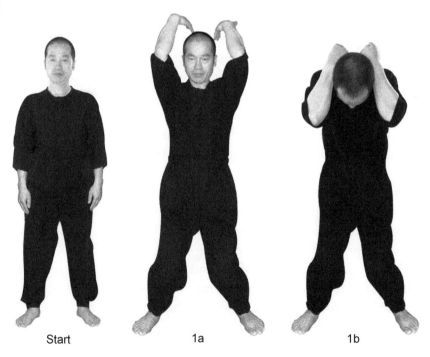

Start   1a   1b

As you become more comfortable, stretch the duration to 15 seconds. After three months of practice, you may try 20 seconds, which means three times per minute.

Make sure to listen to your body. If you feel dizzy, gently kneel or sit and rest until you feel ready to resume practice. If you have discomfort in your neck or spine, reduce the angle of your neck by tilting your head back less.

1. From natural stance, take a deep breath. Exhaling, bend your knees lowering your body, and raise your arms with the palms facing you. Place them next to your head (1a). Make fists, place them beside your neck, and rest your head between them (1b-c).
2. Inhaling, gently tilt your head back, raising your elbows like blossoming lotus petals opening. Lower your knees further to feel the stretch in the torso. After 5-10 seconds, exhaling, return to natural stance. Take a deep breath and repeat.

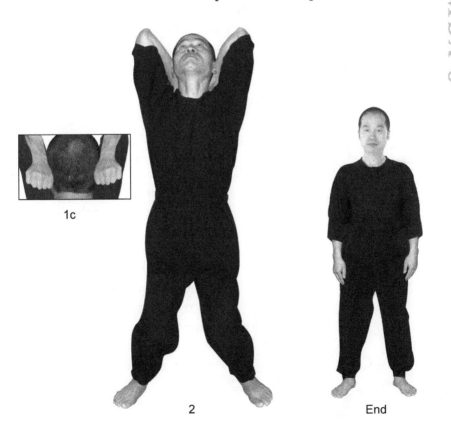

1c

2

End

MBX-8

Focal Points

- The Bubbling Spring (accupoint #1 of the Kidney Meridian, located at the bottom of the foot) is believed to connect the body to and draw in energy from the earth.
- Take up the energy, from the feet to the chest, through a long steady inhalation.
- Keep your knees bent low for stability.
- Look up at the sky and imagine your head is resting between your two fist pillows.
- As you breathe in steadily, feel the stretching sensation rising from the slowly elongating muscles and nerves along the front of the torso.

Self-assessment Criteria

1. Did you feel energy surging up from the feet?
2. Did you feel a soothing sensation in your torso during Head Rest?
3. Did you control your movement at all times?

MBX-8

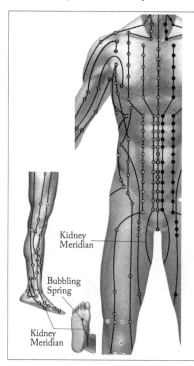

Kidney
Meridian

Bubbling
Spring

Kidney
Meridian

Kidney Meridian

Location: Starts from the small toe and ends at the pericardium.

Function: Interacts with the kidney and communicates with the urinary bladder; connects to the Bladder Meridian and the Pericardium Meridian.

Expected Effects

- Increased relaxation and calmness
- Enhanced sense of balance
- Improved energy circulation

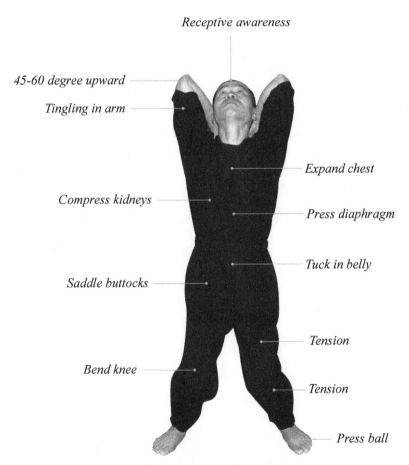

Receptive awareness

45-60 degree upward

Tingling in arm

Expand chest

Compress kidneys

Press diaphragm

Tuck in belly

Saddle buttocks

Tension

Bend knee

Tension

Press ball

Focal Points of Lotus Posture

MBX-8

Ki Energy Paths

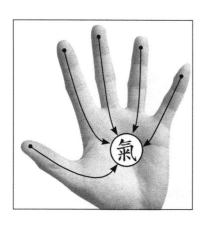

Energy in the body is in constant motion, moving under the radar of our consciousness. Unless the flow is broken we barely notice it. This subconscious business of the body can also be brought to the surface of our consciousness through mindful movement and breathing.

You can practice a simple mindful movement by stretching your fingers wide open. Let's try it. Open both hands as widely as possible. What do you feel? Now relax your hand but remember what you felt to better understand the following explanation.

Whenever you move your body, there is a kind of anti-force that works against it or attempts to return your body to its original condition. For example, when you stretch the muscles of your five fingers, there is a certain resistance that naturally pulls back the muscles in the opposite direction of the stretch. Every action naturally has intrinsic resistance, counterbalancing the change.

Your action is an intentional use of energy; resistance is the body's natural response. When you stretch five fingers, there are five different intentional applications of energy in the direction of the tips of the five fingers. There is also a flow of energy back toward the palm (illustration on opposite page) in the form of resistance. We call both types of invisible energy Ki.

Ki can be collected (photo 1) and redistributed (photo 2). When you raise your arms, resistance is formed in the middle energy center located in the chest area. This resistance draws energy downward. Similarly, when you bend your knees, energy rises from the feet, surging into the lower energy center in the belly area. During inhalation, this energy is collected in the middle and lower energy centers.

When you exhale, the collected energy is redistributed throughout the body (2). Slow exhalation prolongs the redistribution. This type of energy collection and redistribution occurs in the entire body during MBX-12 practice.

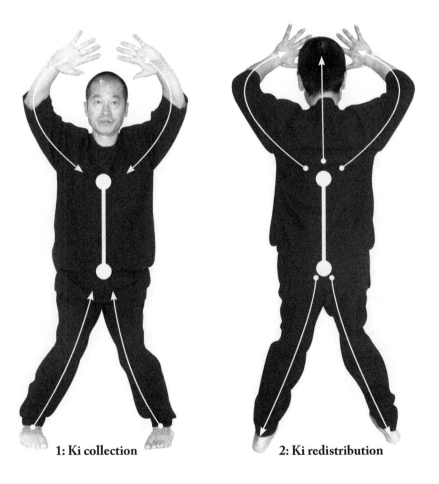

1: Ki collection   **2: Ki redistribution**

9. *Condensing*
Pericardium Meridian

Condensing posture is a diaphragm strengthening exercise. When you inhale, the diaphragm moves down (contraction) sucking air into the lungs. During exhalation, the diaphragm moves upward toward its original position (relaxation).

When you inhale slowly and mindfully and hold your breath for a few seconds, you are holding the diaphragm in a maximally contracted condition, strengthening it. When you exhale slowly and mindfully, controlling every inch of the returning diaphragm, you also strengthen your diaphragm.

Having a strong diaphragm helps you build your inner energy, which is centralized in the middle and lower energy centers. Be aware that your breathing controls and is controlled by the diaphragm.

MBX-9

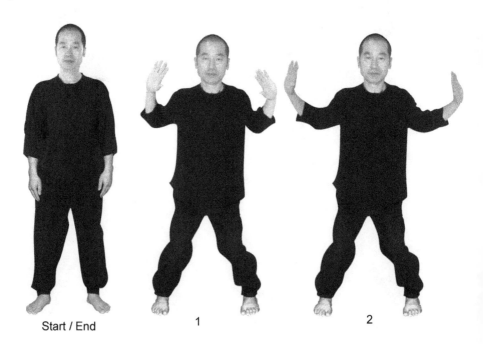

Start / End   1   2

When practicing lateral pushing posture (2), imagine that you are slowly pushing away a wall on each side of you. To do so, you pull the energy from the lower belly to the chest and then to your hands. Remember that your thought directs where your Ki goes, affecting the quality of your performance.

1. From natural stance, place your heels outward and lower your posture. Inhaling slowly and deeply, raise your hands beside your shoulders with your palms sideways. Keep your elbows bent and fingertips upward. *You are collecting the energy in the lower belly.*

2-3. Exhaling, slowly push your palms out to the sides. Push the belly slowly in and release the diaphragm upward. *You are pulling up the energy* to the middle energy center. Hold this posture (3) for 2-3 seconds.

3-4. Exhaling further, lower your hands to the front of the belly (4), and press your palms together to release the remaining air from the lower belly. Inhaling, return to natural stance.

MBX-9

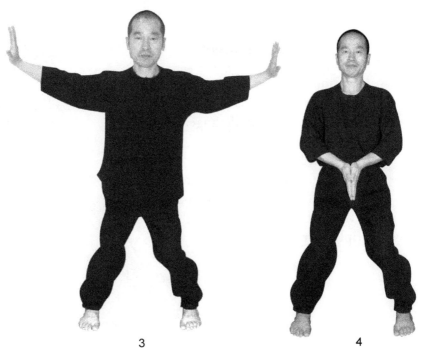

3   4

Focal Points

- Condensing posture increases tension toward the pericardium region and stimulates the Pericardium Meridian.
- During condensing posture (3), exhaling, focus your attention on regulating the contraction of the lower abdomen muscles and relaxation of the rising diaphragm for steady exhalation.
- When you push outward ('Resistance' in the photo on the opposite page), your inner energy in the lower belly is being pushed upward to the chest, and finally being released through the hands. The upward diaphragm movement facilitates the surging energy flow like a piston.
- Keep your middle fingers upright at position 3 to keep the Pericardium Meridian activated.
- During the compression posture (4), exhaling further, contract the belly muscles to push the diaphragm up to the max. Do it gently for safety. Press your palms firmly to argument the compression.
- Strive to develop a sense of control of the diaphragm.

MBX-9

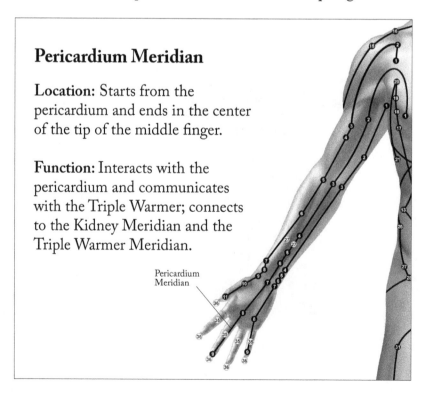

Pericardium Meridian

Location: Starts from the pericardium and ends in the center of the tip of the middle finger.

Function: Interacts with the pericardium and communicates with the Triple Warmer; connects to the Kidney Meridian and the Triple Warmer Meridian.

Pericardium Meridian

Self-assessment Criteria

1. Did you control the belly muscles during breathing?
2. Were you able to sense the movement of the diaphragm ?
3. Did you feel increased awareness in the middle fingers?

Expected Effects

*   Increased sense of balance and physical control
*   Enhanced equanimity and physical composure
*   Boosted energy levels in the torso

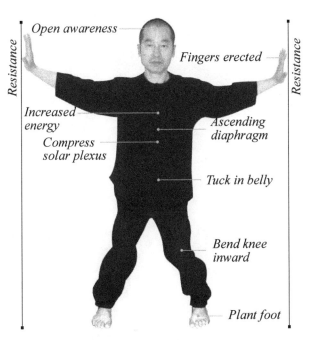

Focal Points of Condensing Posture

BENEFITS OF DEEP BREATHING

Deep breathing enhances the function of the lungs and heart. It vasodilates the blood vessels increasing blood flow and the supply of nutrients to the tissues while eliminating more toxins from the body (compared to regular chest breathing). Consequently, deep breathing refills the reservoir of inner energy and improves the health of the organs and the skin.

MBX-9

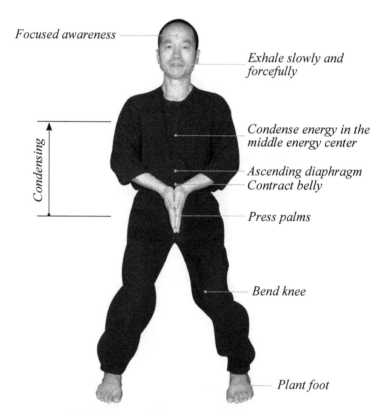

Focused awareness

Exhale slowly and forcefully

Condense energy in the middle energy center

Ascending diaphragm
Contract belly

Press palms

Bend knee

Plant foot

Condensing

Focal Points of Compression Posture

Invisible Precedes Visible

Nature forms and reforms life through the actions and interactions of innate forces. Our body and mind are instruments for those processes. Specifically, the organs are reservoirs and the blood vessels are passages of the life energy we receive from nature.

In Eastern Medicine, this energy is collected in at least three energy centers: the lower energy center in the abdomen, which controls energy production and reproduction; the middle energy center in the chest, which regulates circulation of blood and air; and the upper energy center in the brain, which administers spiritual and cognitive executive functions. These energy centers are connected by meridians, the channels through which the invisible energy flows.

As we know, blood flows through our organs and into tissues for nourishment. Blood flow adapts to the condition of the organs and vessels. Into the organs or vessels that are weak, blood flows weakly. Into the organs with strong inner potential, blood flows forcefully. Blood flow manifests the condition of the vessel through which it flows. If the vessels are damaged, flow is compromised.

In Eastern Medicine, there is the belief that an invisible energy form precedes what is visible. For instance, Ki, an invisible life energy, is followed by the flow of blood, a visible energy carrier. Therefore, what is visible is a manifestation of the action of what is invisible; blood flow is the manifestation of the flow of Ki that precedes it. What we see is what is expressed by the invisible, yet present.

Changes in this invisible energy alter the magnitude, direction, force, and thus the shape of the space that contains both the invisible and visible energy.

Explosive Energy

In sports competition, we often hear explosive shouts when athletes perform explosive movements. Familiar examples are the powerful shouts the Williams sisters make with each tennis stroke or the grunts made by football players when tackling. In martial arts practice, this shout is called kihap or kiai.[1] For centuries, martial artists have been using a controlled breath to create synchronicity of the body and mind.

Martial arts masters can generate extremely powerful forces with their hands and feet. They integrate muscular strength, controlled breath, and mindful focus to unleash the full potential of the body and the mind. When the breath is perfectly timed, it links the flow of energy in the torso and limbs creating a pattern of imperturbable order.

The sudden unleashing of stored energy, accompanied by a sharp exhalation or shout, evokes awe and excitement, which fills the arena with extraordinary life force as athletes push their bodies to the limit. These characteristic shouts also stimulate our senses, allowing us to totally submerge in the world which the player creates. This dynamic integration of mental and physical energy is the foundation of the making of indomitable spirit in us.

---

1   Kihap is Korean term for Ki (vital energy) and Hap (blending). Kiai is Japanese term for Ki (vital energy) and Ai (blending).

Physiologically, an explosive shout has multiple benefits for an athlete. It increases blood flow to the brain and muscles, supplying additional oxygen and glucose to the tissues. It focuses the body's energy, synchronizing the muscles of the limbs and torso with the breath. Psychologically, it builds confidence.

Paradoxically, explosive yelling also relaxes the muscles. The shouting employed by athletes is an intense exhalation. Exhalation stimulates the parasympathetic nervous system which reduces anxiety and physical stimulation. When the body is more relaxed, the muscles gain increased flexibility and range of motion, which in turn increases power.

An illustration drawn from the sport of archery may well explain this phenomenon. If you pull the bow halfway and release, the arrow may fly only 50 feet and drop. But if you pull the bow to the fullest and release, the arrow may fly 200 or 300 feet. The more force that is collected in the bow, the greater distance the arrow can fly. This requires the archer to have knowledge of the potential of his tools (bow and string, and arrow), as well as mindful attention to his movement.

In this example, the string is like the diaphragm. It is a tool that mediates the compression or release of force. The bow is like our body, specifically the lower energy center in the belly, which contains and propels the force. The arrow is like the air that enters and exits the body. The archer's mindful attention is the ability to concentrate on the present moment fully and let go completely.

When the diaphragm, the energy center, and the air are perfectly synchronized during the compressing and releasing stages, a maximal level of energy is produced, resulting in deadly force with an explosive sound.

The take-home message of this explosive energy analogy is that production of maximal force is only possible when maximum stress is unleashed. Stress, a condensed unresolved form of energy, is necessary for release. It is the source for force.

Nasal Breathing

Breathing delivers oxygen to the brain and the muscles, powering and nourishing our mind and body. However, not all breathing is created equal. Scientists have found that blood is oxygenated 10-15% more when you inhale through the nose compared to breathing in through the mouth.

Another little known benefit of inhaling through the nose is the greater concentration of nitric oxide (NO) in the nasal passages. Activated in the nose, NO enters the lungs, relaxing blood vessels, and increasing blood flow. NO is linked to regulation of the cardiovascular, respiratory, nervous, and urogenital systems as well as immune and inflammatory responses. In other words, this colorless, odorless gas can affect the function of your heart, lungs, kidney, urinary tract, brain, and immune system.

NO concentration levels in the breath are as much as fifteen times greater if you create vibration in the nasal cavity, which is believed to mix the air. Chanting, singing, or long slow breathing all create this type of vibration. It's interesting to note that over 2,500 years ago, Buddha developed a deep breathing method for advancing his path to enlightenment that emphasized breathing in through the nose paired with long slow exhalations. Only today is the science becoming available to explain why his method was so advanced.

The Importance of NO and CO₂

Deep breathing impacts pulmonary circulation through nasal breathing and prolonged exhalation. How? Through the body's interaction with nitric oxide and carbon dioxide.

Nitric oxide (NO), known for dilating blood vessels, is abundant in human nasal cavities. So when you breathe in through the nose, your breathing action naturally mixes NO with the air entering the lungs. This dilates the blood vessels in the lungs and expands the bronchioles, small air passages in the lungs which control air distribution. As a result, oxygen transfusion in the lungs increases and your blood becomes more oxygen-rich.

Slow and long exhalations augment the effect. Exhaling slowly for a prolonged period increases the levels of carbon dioxide (CO_2) in the blood. When blood CO_2 increases, oxygen-carrying hemoglobin has a tendency to unload oxygen more readily to surrounding tissues. This accelerates oxygen perfusion in the cells. The result is improved tissue health and increased energy levels.

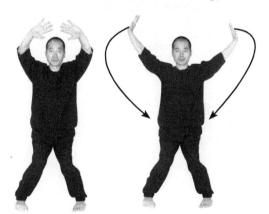

With your hands above your head, fingers wide open, take a few deep breaths, inhaling through your nose (left). This increases NO in your body. Exhale very slowly, lowering your arms as you do (right). This increases oxygen loading in the tissues.

10. Planting

Triple Warmer Meridian

Planting posture strengthens the Triple Warmer area, an imaginary region of the torso that includes the upper warmer (between the glottis and diaphragm), middle warmer (between the diaphragm and navel), and lower warmer (below the navel). This exercise activates the muscles and nerves in the Triple Warmer area by contracting the leg muscles and twisting the arm muscles.

Planting posture is an act of planting a seed of energy in the torso by wringing out the force from the legs and arms, and collecting it in the center of the body. The most beneficial part of the movement is the Low Squat (4), in which you twist the arms with the palms facing outward, lowering your body as close to the ground as possible. This requires strength. You may reduce the intensity of the movement as needed to fit your physical condition.

MBX-10

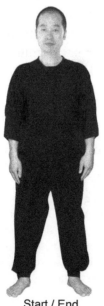

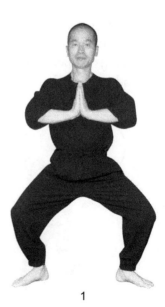

Start / End   1

1. From natural stance, turn your toes outward and lower your posture. Inhale deeply.
2. Exhaling, slowly bend your torso forward, insert your arms between your legs and reach far backward (like someone is pulling your arms).
3. Inhaling, twist your arms and hands inward, so the backs of your hands are facing each other.
4. Exhaling, slowly lower your body as best as you can. Look at the floor. Keep your head and hands horizontal. Hold this position for 3-5 seconds.
5. Inhaling, slowly raise your body to natural stance.

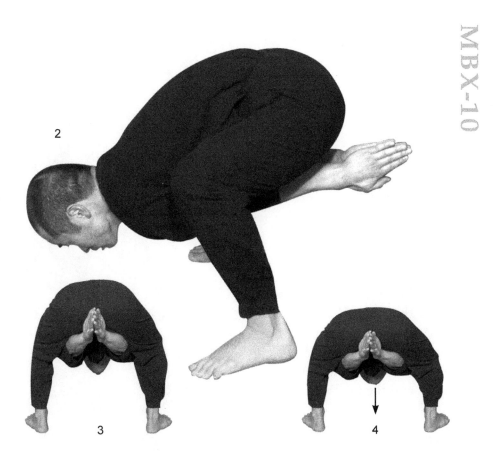

Focal Points

- Done right, Planting posture increases circulation and body heat.
- Move slowly, in the way you feel comfortable. Although this posture appears to be hard to practice, if you do it mindfully, without hurrying, it is no different from looking under the bed for your cat. Along the way, you will find yourself becoming stronger.
- Be open to fresh feelings rising from every inch of your movement. Going one step further, listen to what every fiber in each moving muscle tells you. When you are open to it, you will be able to sense it.
- If you experience cramping or dizziness slowly lower yourself to your knees or lie back and rest.

MBX-10

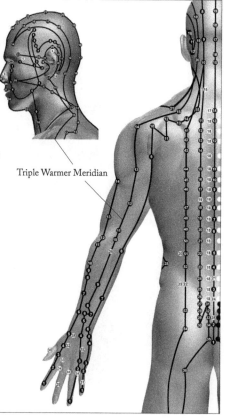

Triple Warmer Meridian

Location: Starts from the lower lateral corner of the fourth fingernail and ends at the lateral side of the eye.

Triple Warmer Meridian

Function: Interacts with the Triple Warmer and communicates with the pericardium; connects to the Pericardium Meridian and the Gallbladder Meridian.

Self-assessment Criteria

1. Did you sense the energy surging from the feet, legs, hips and torso?
2. Did you feel a sense of relief after completion?
3. Did you feel a good sense of centering?

Expected Effects

- Increased sense of balance and strength
- Enhanced circulation
- Boosted inner energy

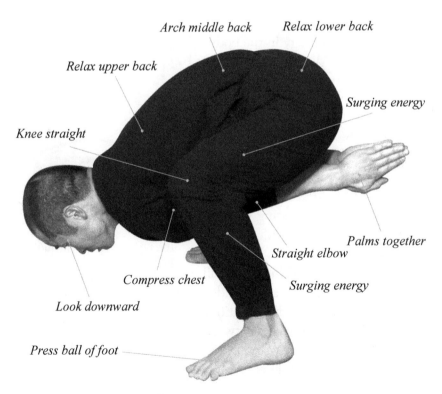

Focal Points of Planting Posture

Triple Warmer: Virtual Organ

The Triple Warmer, a virtual energy space in the torso, is believed to integrate and control the flow of oxygen, blood, nutrients, and excretion. Regarded as one of the six organs in meridian theory, it is the central hub of Ki energy in the body.

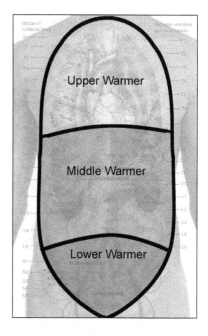

The Triple Warmer has three regions: upper (neck to diaphragm), middle (between diaphragm and navel), and lower (below navel) warmers. The Upper Warmer, consisting of the heart and lungs, is responsible for regulating the circulation of blood and oxygen. The Middle Warmer, consisting of the spleen, stomach, and liver, controls digestion. The Lower Warmer, consisting of the kidneys, small intestine, large intestine, and bladder, regulates excretion. The three sections are divided by the diaphragm between the upper and middle areas and by the navel between the middle and lower regions.

The Upper Warmer, including the heart and lungs, transports oxygen and nutrition. The Middle Warmer, consisting of the spleen, stomach, and liver, is involved in digestion, absorption, and blood production. The Lower Warmer, comprised of the kidney, large intestine, small intestine, and bladder, filters metabolic by-products.

Oxygen Equals Energy

You can increase your energy level in two ways: make more or use less. Our primary method of making more energy is eating food and breaking down its nutrients into usable energy form using oxygen.

You probably already know that oxygen is essential for sustaining our lives. But have you ever given thought to what happens to oxygen once it enters the body?

After entering our body with each breath and traveling through the respiratory and circulatory systems, oxygen is ultimately used to generate a large amount of the energy we need for the body to survive.

Energy for both cognitive function and physical activity is provided via the breakdown of adenosine triphosphate (ATP). Oxygen is a key component in the process of breaking down ATP into usable form. This is why deep slow breathing, which increases oxygen availability, also increases energy production in the brain and muscles.

In addition to increasing energy production through deep breathing, mindfulness practice can reduce the amount of energy burned, which increases energy utility. Studies have shown that during mindful practice such as mediation, our bodies consume less oxygen but paradoxically use the available energy more efficiently.

Breath Control

The diaphragm plays a key role in breath control. When our breathing is short and shallow, the range of diaphragm movement is at a minimum. When we are relaxed, the breath becomes naturally slower and deeper and the range of diaphragm movement enlarges. With practice, you can use your diaphragm to sensitively control the amount, duration, and force of your breath.

The diaphragm is like a passive air bellows. As shown in the illustration on the opposite page, when you open the handles of the bellows, air comes into the flexible bag. During our usual *chest breathing*, as the chest muscles expand, the lungs swell and draw in air, which pushes the diaphragm downward. The chest muscles, however, have limitations in mobilizing the diaphragm further down, partially due to the limited space confined by the thoracic cage.

In deep breathing, called *belly breathing*, the muscles of the abdomen extend outward and pulling the diaphragm much further down than with chest breathing. This enhanced extension of the diaphragm makes additional space for the lungs to swell and bring in more air. In belly breathing, the abdominal muscles function much like the handles of the bellows, creating additional space for air to flow into the expanded lungs. Without the "handles" (the diaphragm and belly muscles), the lungs' capacity to hold air is limited.

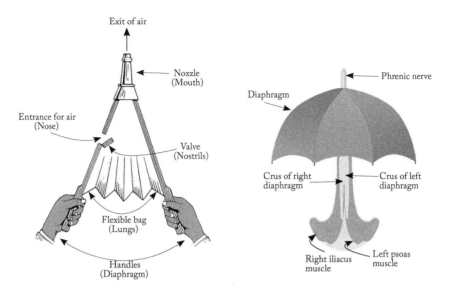

**Symbolic illustrations. Bellows representing inhalation (left).
The umbrella-shaped diaphragm (right).**

Anatomically, the diaphragm is a thin umbrella-shaped muscle (see illustration, above right). When the diaphragm contracts, it pushes downward, increasing the vertical dimension and decreasing the pressure in the chest cavity. This movement allows the lungs to swell.

The diaphragm is directly joined to the anterior (front) abdominal wall in the seam along the rib cage. To gain precision and control over your diaphragm, you need to use the anterior abdominis muscles (belly muscles) to pull the diaphragm downward on inhalation and lift it upward on exhalation. When you extend the abdominal muscles outward during inhalation, your diaphragm contracts (moves downward) to a greater degree, filling your lungs rapidly with a larger volume of air than when you breathe with the chest muscles alone.

During exhalation, you can push additional air out of the lungs by lifting the diaphragm after the chest muscles have completed their contraction. Longer exhalation allows you to expel more carbon dioxide from the body and to unload more oxygen in the cells. In this way, it increases oxygen perfusion in the body.

11. Cradling

Gallbladder Meridian

Cradling posture stretches the lateral sides of body. It activates the Gallbladder Meridian which starts from the side of the eye, circles around the skull, descends on the lateral sides of the torso and legs, and ends at the fourth toenail (see illustration on page 124).

Leftward twist (2) stretches the right side of the body while compressing the other side. The head turns first, then the neck and torso and legs follow. Your feet are planted firmly on the ground, but your knees and hips should be supple enough to accommodate the twist safely. Cradling your torso with your arms creates a sense of unity of the upper body. The lower body provides the leverage and stability for the twist to generate maximum stimulation of the Gallbladder Meridian.

MBX-11

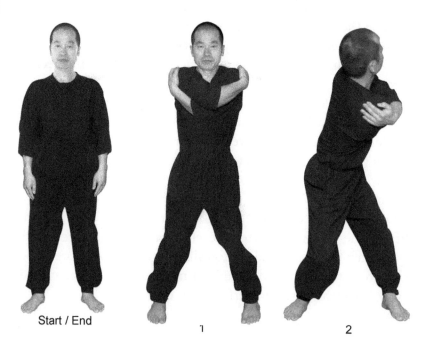

Start / End

1

2

1. From natural stance, place your arms around your body with your hands on the opposite tips of the shoulders. Inhale.
2. Exhaling, slowly turn your head to the left, and then turn your torso. Push your right leg toward your left leg for an additional twist. Hold that position for 3-5 seconds.
3. Inhaling, turn your body to the front.
4. Exhaling, slowly turn your head to the right, and then your torso. Push your left leg toward your right leg for an additional twist. Hold that position for 3-5 seconds.
5. Inhaling, turn your body to the front. Exhaling, return to natural stance.

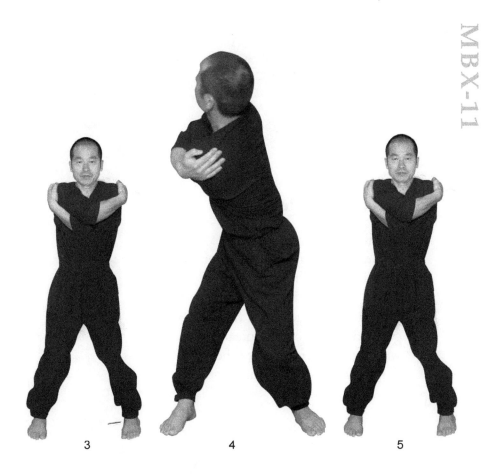

3   4   5

Focal Points

- Cradling is a soothing exercise.
- Slow and progressive mindful turning of the body awakens the vital points along the Gallbladder Meridian. Be aware of the internal changes that occur as you twist.
- Maintain a steady shoulder height during turning, and exhale slowly.
- When you turn your head, scan your eyes along the same horizon to actively engage your attention with visible objects.
- Synchronize your breath and movement. Be one with movement and breath by fulfilling the natural need for out-breath during stretching and in-breath during return to the start position.

MBX-11

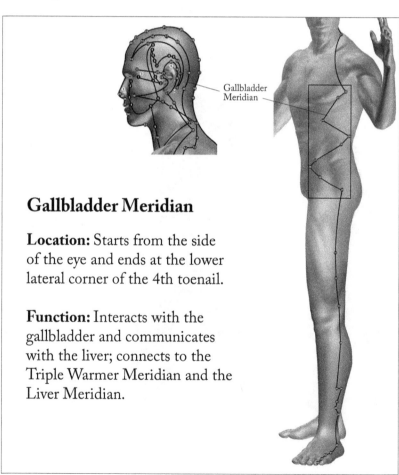

Gallbladder Meridian

Gallbladder Meridian

Location: Starts from the side of the eye and ends at the lower lateral corner of the 4th toenail.

Function: Interacts with the gallbladder and communicates with the liver; connects to the Triple Warmer Meridian and the Liver Meridian.

Three-section Twisting

Twisting starts from the head and neck, then the torso, followed by the lower limbs. Maintain the center of balance while turning.

1. Your head initiates twisting. Rotate your head to the left. Feel contraction on the left side of the neck and stretching on the right side of the skull. Turning the head stimulates meridians of the neck and head.

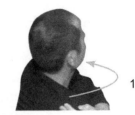

2. Rotate the torso to the left and feel the "wringing" sensation. Torso twisting stimulates the gallbladder and kidney as well as the Gallbladder Meridian.

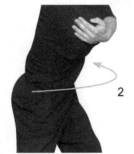

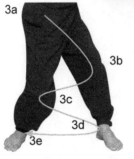

3a-d. As you rotate your hip to the left, the force travels in zigzag via the left and right legs, until it stops at the right foot.

3e. Your feet should be firmly planted to complete the twisting.

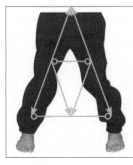

Horse Stance: Secure the bases of your feet. Imagine that filling the space between your feet and the center of gravity with four triangles supporting each other.

Self-assessment Criteria

1. Did you feel stretching and flexing on the sides of your body?
2. Did you experience a soothing effect during or after this exercise?
3. Did you control your movement at all times?

Expected Effects

- Increased sense of comfort
- Enhanced sense of balance
- Increased sense of unity

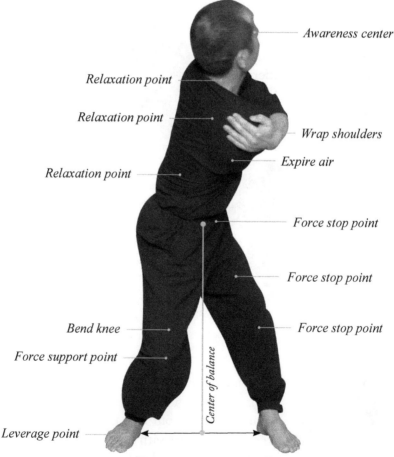

Awareness center

Relaxation point

Relaxation point

Wrap shoulders

Expire air

Relaxation point

Force stop point

Force stop point

Bend knee

Force stop point

Force support point

Center of balance

Leverage point

Focal Points of Cradling Posture

MBX-11

Mind-Body Unity

It isn't possible to empirically prove that the mind and the body are one. But how often have you heard stories of someone experiencing the sense that, 'Yes, I was totally one, and wasn't even conscious of oneness. Nothing!' Perhaps you've had this experience yourself.

We often lose our awareness of the body when we are immersed in an activity like reading a book or playing an instrument. Lost in the flow of total concentration, nothing exists but the doing. You and the book or the guitar vanish. The story or the music and your awareness just are. In that moment, we may say that we are one—that we are a whole—without separation of the mind from the body or the body from the mind.

Our thoughts and feelings belong to the mind; physical sensation belongs to the body. However, physical sensation affects our feelings. Our thoughts, in turn, alter our mental and physical condition. It is nonsensical, then, to say the body and the mind are two separate entities.

On the other hand, it could be argued that they may be arbitrary reflections of each other, instruments of self-identity whose purpose is to verify that we exist.

It is obvious that the mind and the body are not one when we die. The body stays but the mind leaves upon death. Non-living beings have no emotions and thoughts, as far as we know, so we may conclude that the mind no longer exists for them.

When viewed in this paradoxical way, the interactions between the mind and the body are both simple to understand and impossible to fathom.

Stress Buffering

Mindful movement and deep breathing have a buffering effect on stress perception. Generally our body responds to stressful stimuli through hormone secretion by the endocrine system. Working in tandem with the nervous system, the neuro-endocrine system is our primary means of coping with stressors and maintaining balance in our body.

Whether the stress is real or perceived, the body responds in similar ways. The body's stress cascade begins when stressful neural stimuli are perceived by the sensory organs (primarily the eyes and ears). The sensory signals are transmitted to the brain, which activates the sympathetic nervous system, sending out messages to secrete hormones that help the body cope with the stressors. However, regardless of how strong a stimulus may be, if we do not perceive it as a stressor or if we are stress resilient, the impact of the stimulus will be minimized.

No matter what your natural stress tolerance level is, you can improve your stress resilience through taking a mindful approach to stress management. For example, when you intentionally breathe deeply and practice mindful movement, you can feel your heart rate slow. The blood vessels relax and dilate, resulting in increased blood flow and oxygen delivery to every part of your body, including your brain and vital organs. Anxiety lessens and your body's stress response is preempted. The parasympathetic nervous system is stimulated, signaling the sympathetic nervous system to quiet down and buffering the negative impacts of stress.

Sleep Breathing

One traditional method for inducing sleep is rhythmic breathing: breathe, count, and feel the rhythms of your repetitive breathing. Repetition of breath familiarizes you with your own inner rhythm, reducing emotional arousal and helping you slip into sleep.

Method One: Breathe with counting. Breathe in with count one. Breathe out with count two. Keep counting and breathing evenly and rhythmically until you fall asleep.

Method Two: Breathe while counting from one to nine. Breathe in and out with count one. Breathe in and out with count two, continuing in this way up to nine. Then, begin again, repeat the cycle until you fall asleep.

Method Three: Breathe and sense the rhythmic movement of the belly muscles. Belly up and breathe in. Breathe out and belly down. Breathe in at the speed you normally do but use the belly muscles to gently move the air in and out.

Method Four: Breathe and feel the belly. Place your palms gently on the belly. Feel the softness of the belly. Feel the warmth of your palms. Gently, belly up and breathe in. Calmly breathe out and belly down. Focus on how warm your hands and belly are. Feel the softness, warmth, and gentle rhythms of your belly breathing. Keep repeating until you slip into sleep.

12. Unity

Liver Meridian

Unity Posture stimulates the Liver Meridian, which begins from the big toe, ascends through the inner thigh and the lateral torso, and arrives in the liver. This is the most challenging movement in MBX-12 because you stand on a single leg. You also perform multiple movements during the single leg standing: raising your arms sideways and placing one ankle on the knee while bending your standing knee and exhaling. But if you do one movement at a time, very slowly, it becomes a rewarding experience.

The key is developing your internal awareness of the changes in your body so you can better control your body. The irony of controlling is that to control your body, you have to go along with the flow of the body and how you feel in the moment.

Imbalance results from awkwardness. Through repetition, however, you will familiarize your mind with the movements. In time, you will feel more confident, relaxed and balanced. If necessary, you may use a chair to support you and enhance your balance.

MBX-12

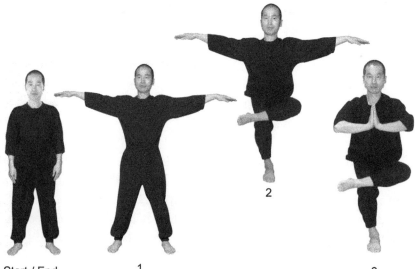

Start / End   1   3

2

1. From natural stance, raise your arms sideways and inhale.
2. Place your left upper ankle above your right knee and gently bend the standing leg. Keep your arms open. Exhale.
3. Inhaling, bring your hands to the front of your chest. Exhaling, gently bend your standing knee. Hold this position for 5-10 seconds.
4. Place your left foot on the ground, raising your arms. Inhale.
5. Place your right upper ankle above your left knee and gently bend the standing leg. Keep your arms open. Exhale.
6. Inhaling, bring your hands to the front of your chest. Exhaling, gently bend your standing knee. Hold this position for 5-10 seconds.
7. Place your right foot on the ground while raising your arms. Inhale.
8. Return to natural stance. Exhale.

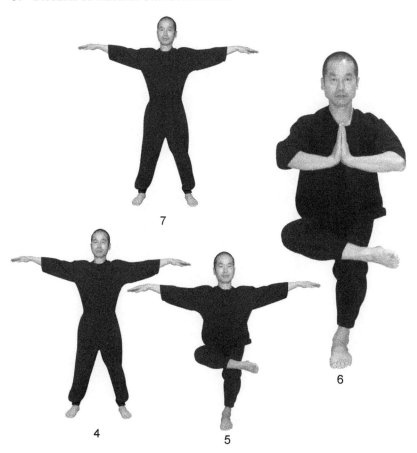

7

6

4

5

Focal Points

- Unity posture connects 4 points in the vertical plane: the foot, the lower, middle and upper energy centers.
- Centering is the key. Stand low and hold your praying hands in the middle of the chest for balance.
- Keep your torso upright and push your hip slightly backward until you feel a stretching sensation in the piriformis muscles that run across the hips.

MBX-12

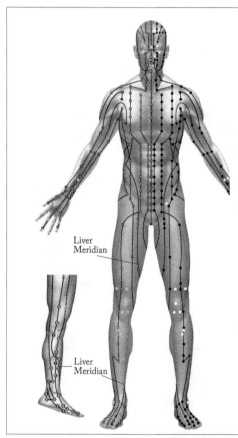

Liver
Meridian

Liver
Meridian

Liver Meridian

Location: Starts from the big toenail and ends at the lungs.

Function: Interacts with the liver and communicates with the gallbladder; connects to the Gallbladder Meridian and the Lung Meridian.

Self-assessment Criteria

1. Did you experience a sense of centering?
2. Did you experience increasing temperature in your body?
3. Did you maintain your balance for at least 3 seconds in position 3 and 6?

Expected Effects

- Increased sense of balance and strength
- Enhanced mental composure
- Increased inner energy

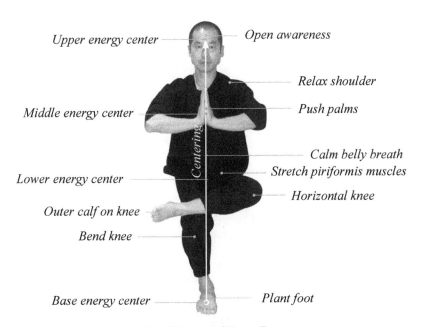

Focal Points of Unity Posture

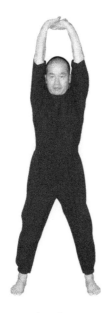

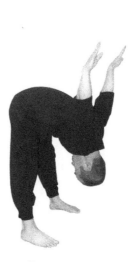

2. Carrier

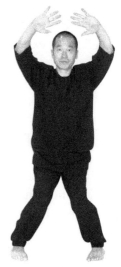

3. Infinity

1. Awakening

MBX-12

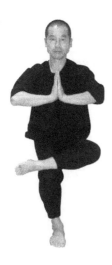

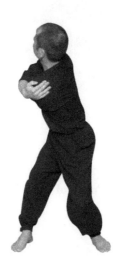

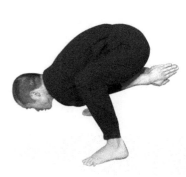

12. Unity

11. Cradling

10. Planting

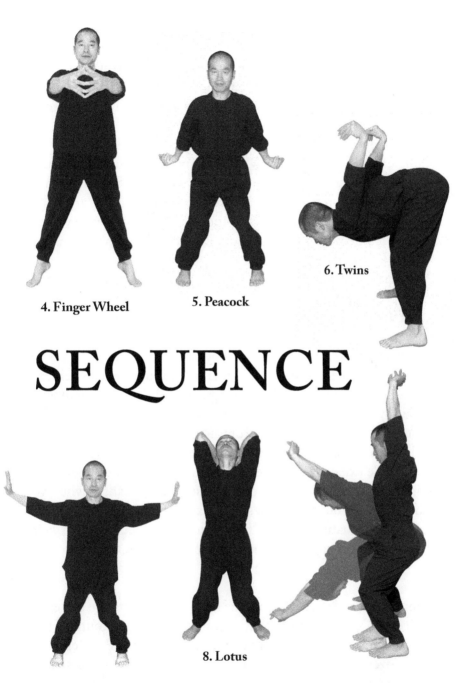

4. Finger Wheel

5. Peacock

6. Twins

SEQUENCE

9. Condensing

8. Lotus

7. Big Bow

How to Link Postures

Once you know how to practice the twelve postures, you can connect them smoothly using transitional movements (see the MBX-12 Sequence on the following pages). The ultimate goal is to connect all twelve postures into one flow in a rhythmic fashion.

The general idea for connecting the postures is that after you complete the sequence of one MBX posture, return to natural stance, then begin the first step of the next MBX posture. So, for example, perform MBX-1, return to natural stance, begin MBX-2 and so on. For an example of how to practice the postures in sequence you can view a video demonstration on Youtube (http://www.youtube.com/watch?v=kWE-m6uQOxo).

Breathing is the linking point. In most cases, you take one in-breath per movement and one out-breath per movement. When you lift your body, breathe in. When you bend or stretch your body, breathe out.

There are postures that employ double inhaling or double exhaling. Double inhaling means inhaling through two movements. For example, for MBX-1 (Awakening posture), you breathe in when you raise your hands above your head, and breathe in further when you stretch your arms at maximum height. This is double inhaling, which helps you expand the capacity of the lungs.

Double exhaling means exhaling through two movements. For example, for MBX-9 (Condensing posture), you exhale when you push your hands out to the sides, then exhale further when you lower your hands to natural stance. This is double exhaling, which helps you improve your capacity to expel toxic gases from the body.

By linking all twelve postures in one flowing sequence, you can either practice MBX-12 in its entirety, or scale it to fit the amount of time you have and the environmental setting you are in. Practicing just a few movements mindfully can stimulate, mobilize, and distribute your inner energy across the body as effectively as practicing the entire set.

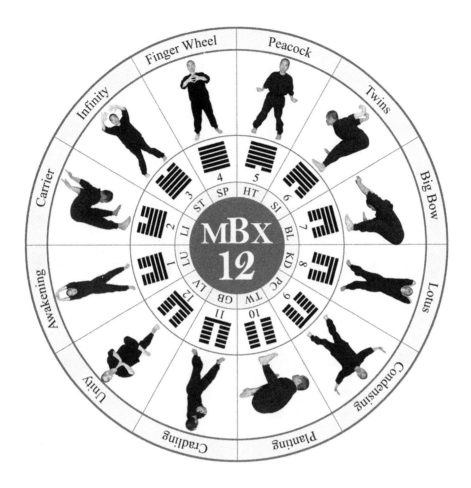

Meaning of MBX-12 Hexagrams

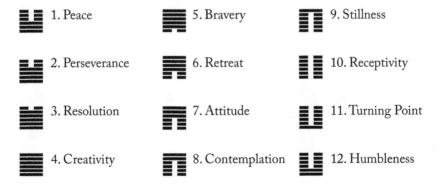

1. Peace

2. Perseverance

3. Resolution

4. Creativity

5. Bravery

6. Retreat

7. Attitude

8. Contemplation

9. Stillness

10. Receptivity

11. Turning Point

12. Humbleness

MBX-12 SEQUENCE

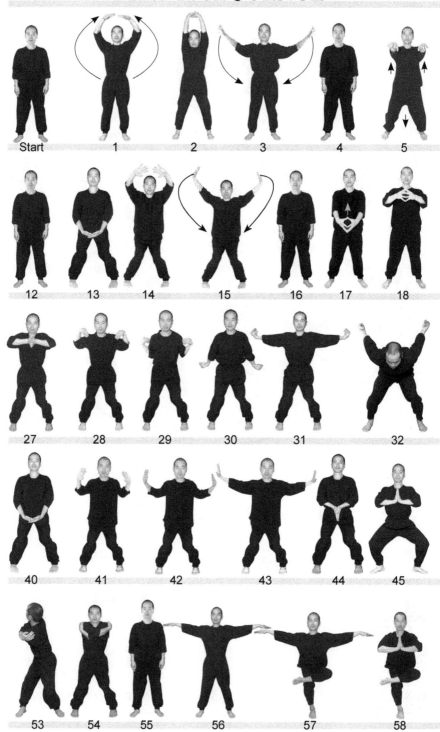

Start 1 2 3 4 5

12 13 14 15 16 17 18

27 28 29 30 31 32

40 41 42 43 44 45

53 54 55 56 57 58

MBX-12 SEQUENCE

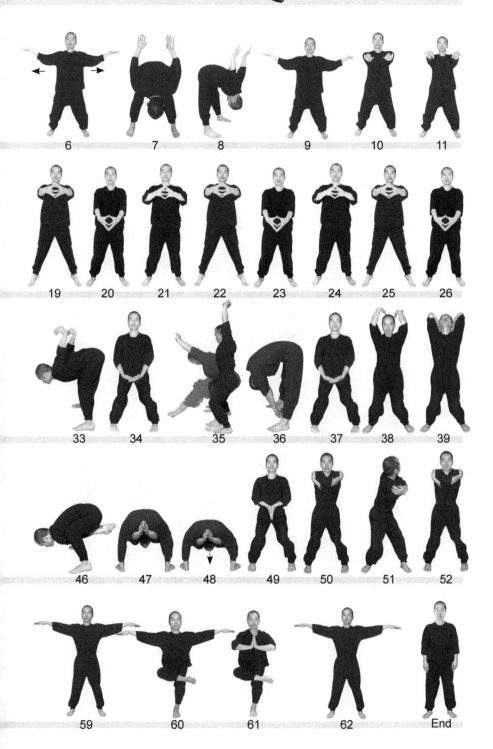

MBX MUDRA

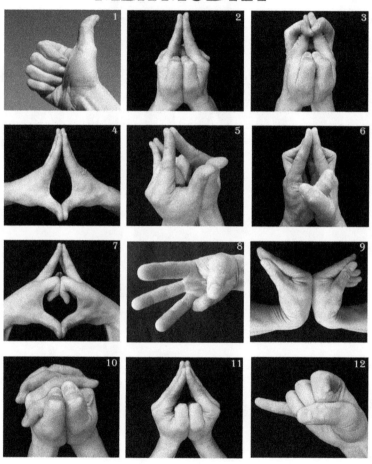

4
MBX Mudra

Mudra is both a symbolic hand movement and a functional way to stimulate the six meridians located in the hands. Mudras are a good way to practice mindfulness when you cannot do full body exercise such as MBX-12.

In the Eastern folk medicine, the hand is believed to be a miniature of the human body. The middle finger corresponds to the head and torso, the index and ring fingers to the hands, the thumb and little finger to the feet. More importantly, the hands are energy terminals and transition points, receiving energy from the organs and returning energy to the organs via the meridians.

Energy that flows from the center of the body to the terminals follows yin meridians, which run inside of the arm toward the fingertips. In MBX Mudra practice, we call this terminal energy flow (TEF). Central energy flow (CEF), on the other hand, refers to terminal energy flowing to the center of the body. CEF follows yang meridians, which run outside of the arm from the fingertips toward the torso. For Yin meridians, inhale while pressing the fingers to expand energy to the fingers. For Yang meridians, exhale while pressing the fingers to send energy to the center.

Each mudra stimulates specific meridians and, in turn, specific organs. Pressing, stretching, or twisting the fingers as described in the mudra instructions activates the corresponding meridians in the hand and affects energy flow in the corresponding organ(s).

THE HAND IS A MINIATURE OF THE BODY

According to Eastern folk medicine, the hand is regarded as a miniature of the human body. The middle finger corresponds to the head and torso, the index and ring fingers to the hands, the thumb and little finger to the feet. Conceptually, when you stimulate the hand meridians through MBX Mudra practice, you are stimulating the entire body.

As illustrated below, there are six meridians in the hand: three yin meridians on the inside and three yang meridians on the outside. Through these meridian networks, each finger is linked to a specific corresponding organ.

For a balanced experience, always practice MBX Mudra using both hands simultaneously. When done correctly, Mudra practice stimulates the left and right sides of the brain, widens the field of your awareness, and creates mental and physical equilibrium giving you a calming feeling.

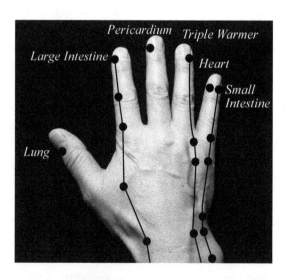

There are 6 meridians in the hand: 3 inside in the palm and 3 on the back of the hand. The 3 inside channels are yin (passive) meridians and the 3 outside are yang (active) meridians.

Warm Up: Hand Mirrors Body

Stretching the fingers open wide stimulates the six meridians present in the hands and along the arms as well as the nerve connections to the lungs, heart, large intestine, and small intestine. Gently opening and closing both hands is a good way to warm-up the hands and awaken your inner energy channels prior to practicing MBX Mudra exercises.

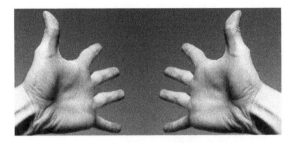

Gently open your hands as wide as possible, spreading your fingers and thumb five to ten times before beginning MBX Mudra practice.

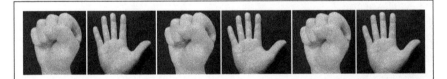

Relaxation Between Exercises. Stretching the muscles in the hand is no different from stretching any other muscles. If overdone, it may cause pain or discomfort in your hands and forearms.

You can prevent this by clenching and opening your hands a few times between exercises, or gently shaking your hands.

1. *Thumbs Up*
Lung Meridian

Stretching your thumbs up stimulates the Lung Meridian. Take a deep breath while stretching. Breathe out while releasing. This mudra helps you refresh your vigor and uplift your energy levels.

MBX MUDRA 1

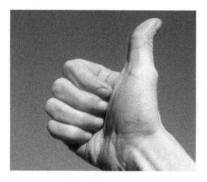

1. Clench your fists. Raise both arms and hands in front of you.
2. Inhaling deeply, stretch your thumbs maximally. Raise your hands to chest level and expand your chest. Feel the energy flowing from the lungs to the thumbs.
3. With your thumbs up, exhale slowly. Feel the energy returning to the lungs. Repeat 5-10 times.

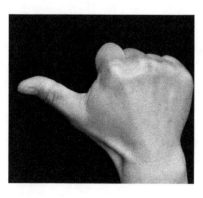

Change positions:
You may alter the direction or weight of your hand. For example, turn your thumb inward or outward, or place your hand above your head or below your belt level. Do it slowly so that you can sense minute changes in the intensity of the activation.

Energy Flow Direction: Terminal*

Terminal energy flow (TEF) is energy that flows from the center of the body to the terminals, following yin meridians.

2. Diamond Hands
Lung Meridian

Diamond Hands mudra stimulates the Lung Meridian along the inner arc of the thumbs. Gently press the fingers, inhaling. Expand your lungs and stretch the thumbs. Exhaling, let go.

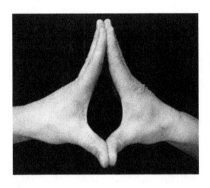

1. Place all the corresponding fingertips against each other.
2. Inhaling, gently press the fingers together. Feel the energy flowing from the lungs to the thumbs.
3. Exhaling, relax the fingers while keeping the fingertips touching. Feel the energy leaving the hands.

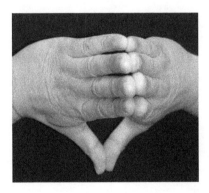

Focal Point:
Give extra pressure at the contact point of the thumbs. Look down at the contact point for visual concentration. Inhaling, increase the pressure and move your hands gently into the chest. Exhaling, reduce the pressure and gently release the hands.

Energy Flow Direction: Terminal

3. *Triad*

Large Intestine Meridian

Triad mudra stimulates the Large Intestine Meridian, which runs along the upper outer index fingers. Gently press the index fingers and contract the buttocks while exhaling. Release while inhaling.

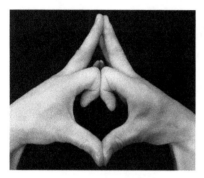

1. Put your palms together.
2. Bend your index fingers. Inhale.
3. Exhaling, press the index fingers as shown and contract the muscles in the pelvic floor.
4. Inhaling, release the tension while keeping the fingers touching. Feel the relaxing sensation in the buttocks.

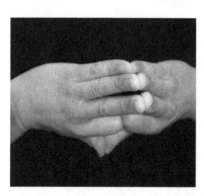

Centralizing Energy
When you press the index fingers, focus on the inner upper edges where the Large Intestine meridian is located. Begin with gentle pressure. Do three things simultaneously for Triad mudra: press the index fingers, contract the buttocks, and exhale. Those three actions condense energy into the Large Intestine area.

Energy Flow Direction: Central*

Central energy flow (CEF) is energy that flows from the terminals to the center of the body, following yang meridians.

MBX MUDRA 3

4. *Interwoven Fingers*
Large Intestine Meridian

Interwoven Fingers mudra stimulates the Large Intestine Meridian when you press the vital points on the upper index fingers. Gently press the index fingers and contract the buttocks while exhaling. Release while inhaling.

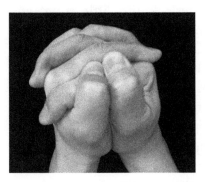

1. Interlock the fingers. Inhale.
2. Exhaling, firmly press the first index finger with both thumbs, contracting the pelvic floor muscles.
3. Inhaling, relax the hands and buttocks.
4. Interlock the fingers, placing the other index finger closest to the thumb and repeat 1 through 3.

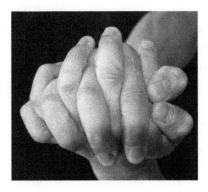

Integrative Effects:
Immediately after Triad mudra (mudra #3), perform Interwoven Fingers. Both mudras stimulate the Large Intestine meridian. For integrative effects, you may alternate these two techniques in the following order: Triad > Interwoven Fingers (right index press) > Triad > Interwoven Fingers (left index press).

Energy Flow Direction: Central

5. Heavenly Fingers
Heart Meridian

Heavenly Fingers mudra stimulates the inner tip of the little finger, the end of the Heart Meridian. Inhaling, press your little fingers against the area near the opposite knuckle. Imagine the energy from the heart arriving at the fingertips.

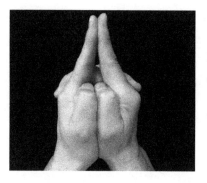

1. Interlock the little, ring, and middle fingers.
2. Keep the index fingers straight.
3. Bend the thumbs as shown. Exhale.
4. Inhaling, squeeze the little fingers against the back of the opposite hand as hard as you can.
5. Exhaling, relax.

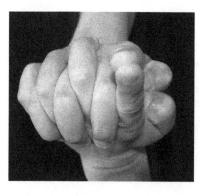

Big Force on Little Finger:
When you inhale and press the little fingers, move your hands gently closer to your body. Imagine you are sending energy from the heart to the little fingers. Feel the force at your fingertips. Exhaling, let your hands move gently away from the body.

Energy Flow Direction: Terminal

MBX MUDRA 5

6. *Benevolence*

Heart Meridian

Benevolence mudra stimulates the ending accupoint of the Heart Meridian, located at the tip of the little finger. This is a Yin meridian which runs outward from the heart. Inhale while pressing the fingers to extend the energy to the terminal.

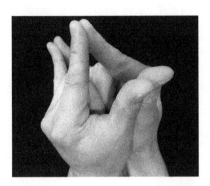

1. Bend the ring and middle fingers, facing each other.
2. Press the tips of the little fingers and index fingers.
3. Keep the thumbs straight.
4. Inhaling, firmly press the tips of the little fingers together.
5. Exhaling, relax.

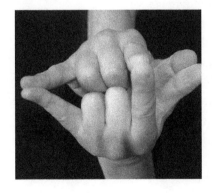

With All Your Heart:
The heart is where our feelings unite. When you gently but firmly press the little fingers, close your eyes and bring your hands close to your chest. Imagine that the energy from the heart connects with the smallest tips of the little fingers. With all your heart, send warm energy to the little terminals. It unites you.

Energy Flow Direction: Terminal

7. Loyalty
Small Intestine Meridian

Loyalty mudra stimulates the Small Intestine Meridian, which is Yang-type. Energy runs from the outer little fingertip to the front of the ear. As you exhale, increase the pressure and feel the flow.

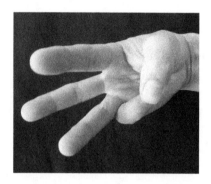

1. Press the little fingernail with the tip of your thumb. Inhale.
2. Exhaling, increase the resistance of the little finger against the thumb.
3. Inhaling, release the tension.

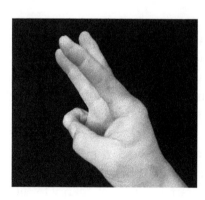

Breath Massage:
When you contract the belly muscles and slowly breathe out, it has an effect of gently massaging the organs, especially the small intestine. Exhalation releases the intestines. While practicing Loyalty mudra, close your eyes and feel the gentle massage work of the belly muscles on your intestine as the intensity on the little fingertips increases.

Energy Flow Direction: Central

8. *Acceptance*
Small Intestine Meridian

Acceptance mudra stimulates the energy channel connected to the small intestine. Exhaling, press the fingertips together, focusing primarily on gently pressing the outer edge of the little fingers.

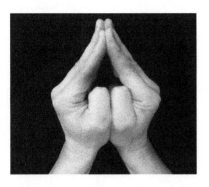

1. Put the palm heels together.
2. Bend the little fingers and thumbs so they are touching along the outer edges. Inhale.
3. Exhaling, increase pressure on the index, middle and ring fingertips, then on the little fingers.
4. Inhaling, relax.

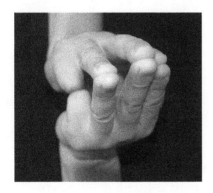

Mindful Awareness:

One way to improve your mindfulness is to be aware of your whole self by focusing on the sensation in a particular area of the body. In Acceptance mudra, you may practice spreading the initial attention on the little fingers to the arms and torso, then to the entire body. Like in prayer, your sensation becomes one with your body and encircles you as a whole.

Energy Flow Direction: Central

9. *Intelligence*
Pericardium Meridian

Intelligence mudra stimulates the Pericardium Meridian which is associated with gut feelings and self-confidence. This exercise also induces a calming effect and stimulates the imagination.

MBX MUDRA 9

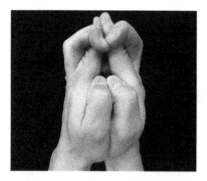

1. Cross your middle fingers over your index fingers.
2. Interlock the little and ring fingers.
3. Bend the thumbs.
4. Inhaling, pull the middle fingers toward the base of the index fingers. Feel the central energy flowing to the fingers.
5. Exhaling, relax.

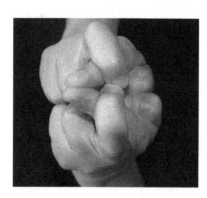

Brain and Finger Talk:
Stimulating the fingers stimulates the brain. Intelligence mudra activates the brain through the vagus nerve and promotes a soothing, calming sensation. When you are entangled with complex brain work, take a deep breath in and practice Intelligence mudra. It stimulates the part of the brain that is responsible for imagination and creativity.

Energy Flow Direction: Terminal

10. Calm Hands
Pericardium Meridian

Calm Hands mudra brings your attention to the tip of the inner middle fingertips. It stimulates the Pericardium Meridian which is Yin-type and carries the energy from the center to the terminal.

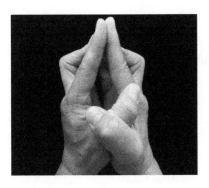

1. Put your palms together.
2. Interlock your thumbs. Exhale.
3. Inhaling, increase pressure on the tips of the middle fingers. Feel the energy concentrating at the middle fingertips originating from the center of the torso.
4. Exhaling, relax.

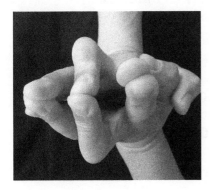

The Heart Brain:
Structurally the middle finger represents the head of human body. Energetically it is associated with the heart. By stimulating the middle finger, you link the heart and the brain. To feel the connection, bring your hands closer to the heart when you press them while inhaling.

Energy Flow Direction: Terminal

MBX MUDRA 10

11. Goose Head
Triple Warmer Meridian

Goose Head mudra stimulates the Triple Warmer meridian that runs along the ring finger. Bend your wrist into the shape of goose head and gently role the backs of the hands against each other.

MBX MUDRA 11

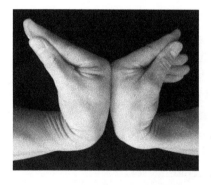

1. Put the backs of the hands together, fingers facing upward, like goose heads. Align the back of the hands so that the outer upper side of the ring fingers match. Inhale.
2. Exhaling, gently press the backs of the hands by lowering them.
3. Inhaling, relax.

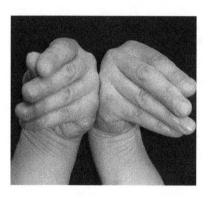

Accidental Findings:

Goose Head is a mudra that you can vary to fit your body type. Experiment with various angles and intensities while practicing. You may practice it with your hands vertically upward or downward. Or practice both methods alternately.

Energy Flow Direction: Central

12. Attitude

Triple Warmer Meridian

Attitude mudra stimulates the Triple Warmer meridian, an imaginary organ of the body that functions like an energy control center, regulating the consumption, distribution, and disposal of food and other energy resources.

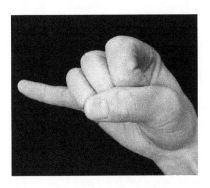

1. Bend the thumb, index, middle and ring fingers.
2. Pressing the three fingernails with the thumb, inhale.
3. Exhaling, increase the resisting force of the ring finger against the thumb. Feel the energy flowing from the finger to the torso.
4. Inhaling, relax.

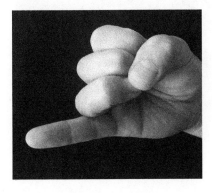

Complementary Effect:
When you create tension in the hand by pressing the ring finger against the thumb, a relaxed sensation arises in the Triple Warmer. When you release the tension in the fingers, there is a complementary sensation in the Triple Warmer of a renewed tension as it returns to its original condition.

Energy Flow Direction: Central

MBX MUDRA 12

Reflection
Cool Down

Reflection mudra is for soothing the six meridian channels in your hands. Gently press the fingertips and release. Shift the intensity of pressure along the fingers in a wave-like motion, rolling the fingertips against each other to create a soft sensation. Experiment with different ways of soothing the fingers with this mudra. Inhale and exhale freely during reflection.

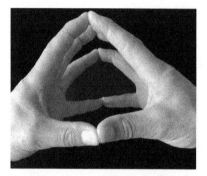

1. Put the fingertips gently together.
2. Be aware of the fresh feeling of contact at each fingertip.
3. Breathe in and out softly and let your mind drift as you roll your hands gently toward and away from your body.

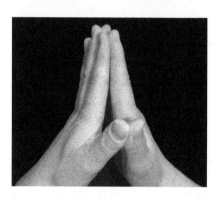
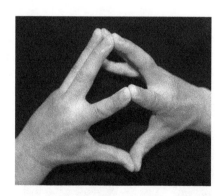

Gentle practice of Reflection mudra may elicit a sense of togetherness. Roll your hands gently around with the fingertips touching. Feel the softly moving finger joints adapting and readapting to the changing pressure and direction.

Result: soothing and calming effects

5
Wellness Applications

Each MBX-12 posture activates a specific meridian and boosts inner energy circulation. At the same time, each posture stimulates multiple meridians because the network of the human body is closely integrated. Stimulation of one part of the body affects other areas of the body, creating a rippling effect. This is both positive and desirable.

As a result of this integrative effect, many people find that activating specific meridians can decrease anxiety and headaches, and improve a sense of balance.

In the following pages, you will find six postures that stimulate the meridians commonly associated with improvement in anxiety, four postures for balance, and three postures for headache.

Anxiety

Anxiety results from a perceived stressor or a break in the synchronization between your internal rhythm and your external environment. For example, an external stressor is disrupting your biorhythms, causing changes in the physiological response of your body such as rising blood pressure, increased urination, elevated glucose production and reduced digestive function. The following exercises have a soothing affect by targeting the associated meridians.

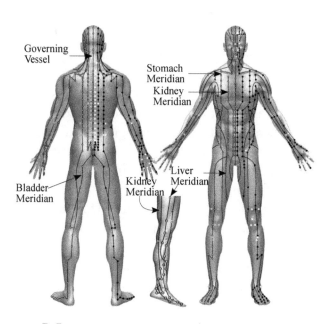

Meridians for Anxiety

Meridian	Accupoint	Exercise
Bladder Meridian	BL 10-25, 36-50, 65-67	Big Bow
Kidney Meridian	KI 1-6	Lotus
Stomach Meridian	ST 44-45	Infinity
Governing Vessel	GV 11, 12	Carrier
Liver Meridian	LV 1-3	Unity
Triple Warmer	TW 18-23	Planting

BIG BOW

1. From natural stance, inhaling, stretch your arms as high as you can with one hand overlapping the other and the palms facing upward.
2. Exhaling, slowly lower your stance.
3. Inhaling, slowly bend your body forward and reach your hands out to the front until your hands reach the floor (3a-3b).
4. Exhaling, lift your hip slightly and stretch your arms further forward (or place your hands on the floor). Feel the release in the lower back. This is the key movement in this posture for reducing anxiety.
5. Inhaling, very slowly arch your back and bring your body up to natural stance.

Perform slowly and mindfully to normalize ki flow of bladder meridian, which influences blood pressure.

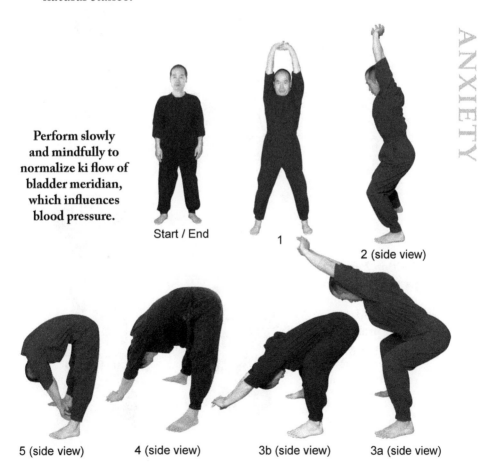

Start / End

1

2 (side view)

5 (side view)   4 (side view)   3b (side view)   3a (side view)

ANXIETY

LOTUS

1. From natural stance, take a deep breath. Exhaling, bend your knees lowering your body, and raise your arms with the palms facing you. Place them next to your head (1a). Make fists, place them beside your neck, and rest your head between them (1b).
2. Inhaling, gently tilt your head back, raising your elbows like blossoming lotus petals opening. Lower your knees further to feel the stretch in the torso. After 5-10 seconds, exhaling, return to natural stance. Take a deep breath and repeat.

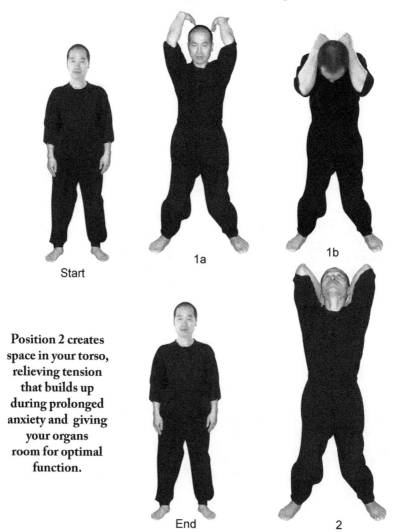

Start

1a

1b

Position 2 creates space in your torso, relieving tension that builds up during prolonged anxiety and giving your organs room for optimal function.

End

2

ANXIETY

INFINITY

1. From natural stance, point your heels outward and bend your knees. Place your open hands in front of your belly with palms facing upward. Exhale

2. Inhaling, raise your hands above your head with your fingers wide open. Pause for 3 seconds. Exhaling very slowly, bend your knees slightly. In the same position, inhale quickly and deeply; then exhale very slowly.

3. Inhaling deeply, push your hands upward to maximum extension (3a). Slowly exhale while lowering your hands sideways to your hips (3b). End in natural stance.

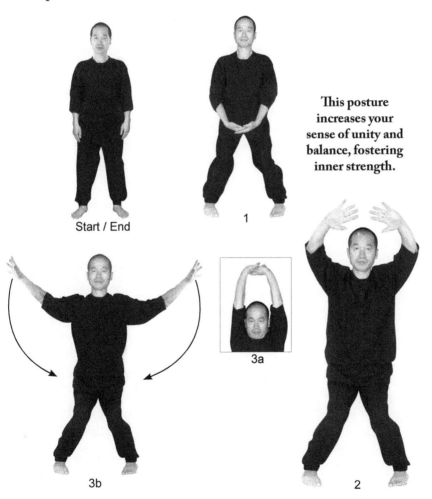

Start / End

1

This posture increases your sense of unity and balance, fostering inner strength.

3a

3b

2

ANXIETY

CARRIER

1. From natural stance, inhaling, slowly bend your knees and raise your arms upward, with your elbows straight and wrists relaxed in front of you (1).
2. Inhaling further, open your arms to the side, rotating the arms until the palms are facing upward (2).
3. Exhaling, rotate your arms inward until your palms are facing the ground. Gently lower your head and raise your arms vertically behind your back (3).
4. Inhaling, straighten the knees. Exhaling, shift your weight to your heels and lower your head a bit (4). Breathe normally in this position. Feel the tension in your hamstrings and the release of the pelvic floor. This posture relaxes the muscles of the rectum, the end of the large intestine.
5. Inhaling, slowly raise your body, rotating the arms outward until they are extended to your side with the palms facing upward (5). Keep the elbows slightly bent .
6. Exhaling, bring your arms to the front slowly, with the palms facing upward (6).
7. Inhaling, rotate the arms inward quickly (7). Gently lower the arms and exhale. End in natural stance.

ANXIETY

Carrier posture reduces the burden of standing upright. Blood flow to the head increases during forward bending while the intestines move toward the solar plexus releasing pressure in the pelvic region. Carrier posture also stimulates the Governing Vessel, which runs along the midline of the back, ascending to the head and descending to the face. As a result, this posture relaxes the organs and refreshes the brain, reducing the negative effects of anxiety.

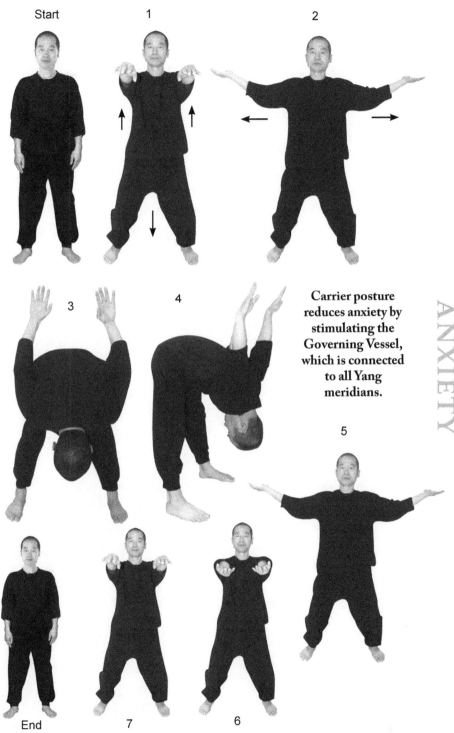

Start   1   2

3   4

Carrier posture reduces anxiety by stimulating the Governing Vessel, which is connected to all Yang meridians.

5

End   7   6

ANXIETY

Uɴɪᴛʏ

1. From natural stance, raise your arms sideways and inhale.
2. Place your left upper ankle above your right knee and gently bend the standing leg. Keep your arms open. Exhale.
3. Inhaling, bring your hands to the front of your chest. Exhaling, gently bend your standing knee. Hold this position for 5-10 seconds.
4. Place your left foot on the ground, raising your arms. Inhale.
5. Place your right upper ankle above your left knee and gently bend the standing leg. Keep your arms open. Exhale.
6. Inhaling, bring your hands to the front of your chest. Exhaling, gently bend your standing knee. Hold this position for 5-10 seconds.
7. Place your right foot on the ground while raising your arms. Inhale.
8. Return to natural stance. Exhale.

Unity posture builds inner strength. Your physical attention is brought to the standing foot; your mental focus is on your hands in front of the chest. These two foci are linked by your awareness of the whole. The meditative holistic awareness that results reduces inner conflicts of the mind and body, which helps you experience oneness: absence of conflicts or anxiety.

ANXIETY

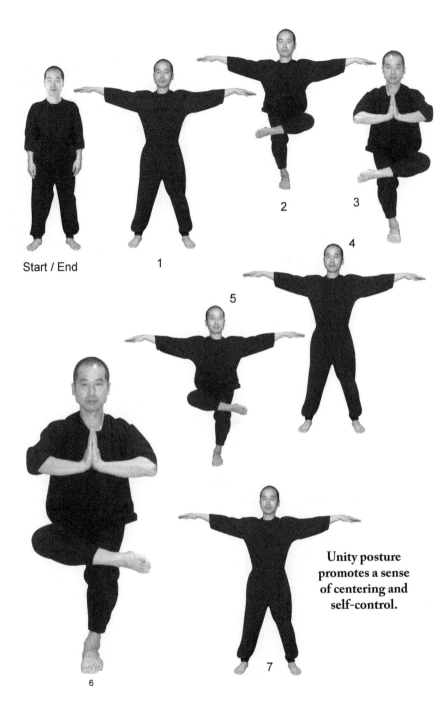

Start / End   1

2   3

4

5

ANXIETY

**Unity posture
promotes a sense
of centering and
self-control.**

6   7

PLANTING

1. From natural stance, turn your toes outward and lower your posture. Inhale deeply.
2. Exhaling, slowly bend your torso forward, insert your arms between your legs and reach far backward (like someone is pulling your arms).
3. Inhaling, twist your arms and hands inward, so the backs of your hands are facing each other.
4. Exhaling, slowly lower your body as best as you can. Look at the floor. Keep your head and hands horizontal. Hold this position for 3-5 seconds.
5. Inhaling, slowly raise your body to natural stance.

ANXIETY

Planting posture stimulates the Triple Warmer meridian and strengthens your body by using a low center of gravity. Like a farmer who plants a seed into the ground in the spring and harvests in the fall, you are sowing your energy into the earth, connecting it, and bringing it up into you. This connection to the power of Mother Earth provides you with a profound sense of inner strength. Only those who sow can reap it. This posture enhances blood circulation and the detoxification process, which promotes the removal of stress by-products in the body.

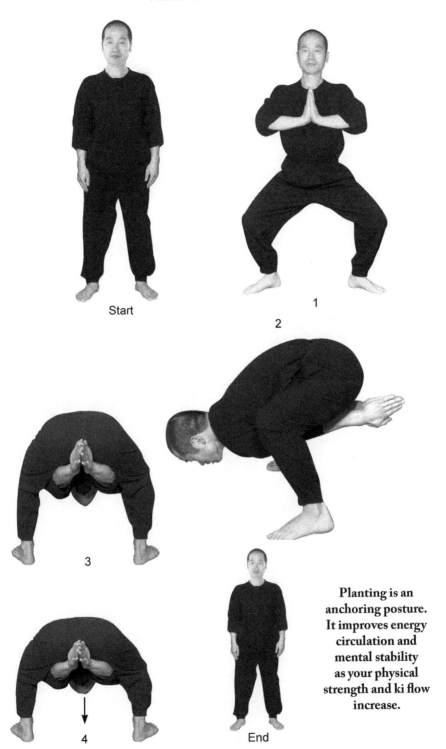

Start

1

2

3

4

End

ANXIETY

Planting is an anchoring posture. It improves energy circulation and mental stability as your physical strength and ki flow increase.

Balance

Balance is a fundamental component of standing, walking, running and daily functional activities. Good balance results from well-coordinated regulation of the sense organs and muscular strength. MBX postures awaken the sense organs such as the proprioceptors and vestibular system. MBX also enhances a sense of awareness of your energy flow, your ability to control your body in transitions, and your ability to maintain equilibrium.

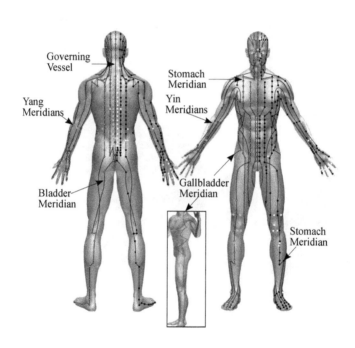

MERIDIANS FOR BALANCE

Meridian	Accupoint	Exercise
Gallbladder Meridian	GB 34, 37, 38, 42	Cradling
Kidney Meridian	KI 2, 9	Lotus
Governing Vessel	GV 2-14	Twins
Stomach Meridian	ST 26-32, 36-45	Infinity

CRADLING

1. From natural stance, place your arms around your body with your hands on the opposite tips of the shoulders. Inhale.
2. Exhaling, slowly turn your head to the left, and then turn your torso. Push your right leg toward your left leg for an additional twist. Hold that position for 3-5 seconds.
3. Inhaling, turn your body to the front.
4. Exhaling, slowly turn your head to the right, and then turn your torso. Push your left leg toward your right leg for an additional twist. Hold that position for 3-5 seconds.
5. Inhaling, turn your body to the front. Exhaling, return to natural stance.

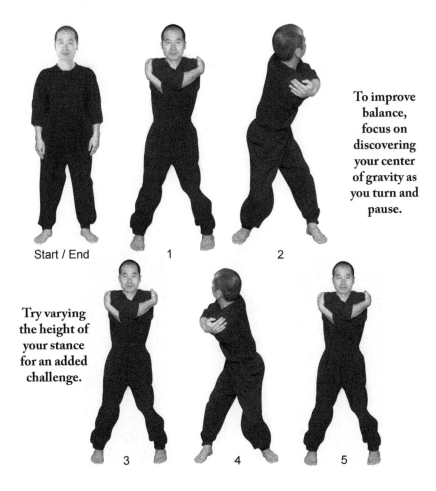

Start / End   1   2

To improve balance, focus on discovering your center of gravity as you turn and pause.

Try varying the height of your stance for an added challenge.

3   4   5

BALANCE

LOTUS

1. From natural stance, take a deep breath. Exhaling, bend your knees lowering your body, and raise your arms with the palms facing you. Place them next to your head (1a). Make fists, place them beside your neck, and rest your head between them (1b).
2. Inhaling, gently tilt your head back, raising your elbows like blossoming lotus petals opening. Lower your knees further to feel the stretch in the torso. After 5-10 seconds, exhaling, return to natural stance. Take a deep breath and repeat.

BALANCE

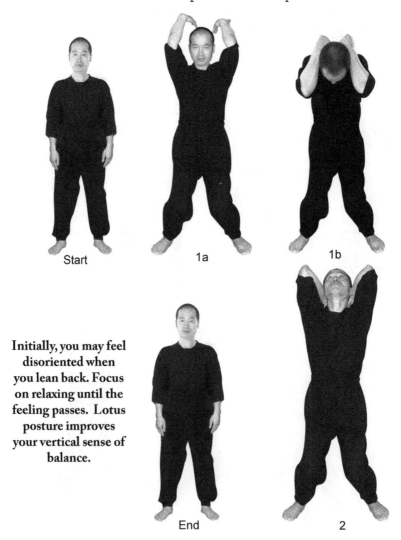

Start   1a   1b

Initially, you may feel disoriented when you lean back. Focus on relaxing until the feeling passes. Lotus posture improves your vertical sense of balance.

End   2

TWINS

1. From natural stance, place your heels outward and bend your knees. This is the ending position of Peacock posture (MBX-5). Exhale.
2. Inhaling, raise your arms to shoulder height on your sides.
3. Exhaling, slowly bend your body forward and raise your arms backward while rotating your arms inward.
4. Inhaling, straighten your legs. Exhaling, shift your weight to your toes, raising your arms backward vertically and lowering your head as much as you can while looking at the ground. Hold for 5-10 seconds while breathing normally.
5. Slowly raise your body and return to natural stance.

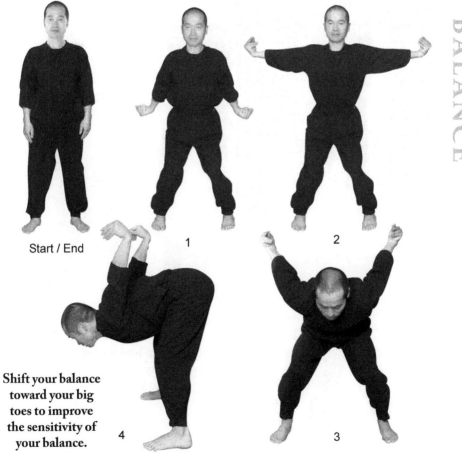

Start / End

1

2

Shift your balance toward your big toes to improve the sensitivity of your balance.

4

3

BALANCE

INFINITY

1. From natural stance, point your heels outward and bend your knees. Place your open hands in front of your belly with palms facing upward. Exhale

2. Inhaling, raise your hands above your head with your fingers wide open. Pause for 3 seconds. Exhaling very slowly, bend your knees slightly. In the same position, inhale quickly and deeply; then exhale very slowly.

3. Inhaling deeply, push your hands upward to maximum extension (3a). Slowly exhale while lowering your hands sideways to your hips (3b). End in natural stance.

BALANCE

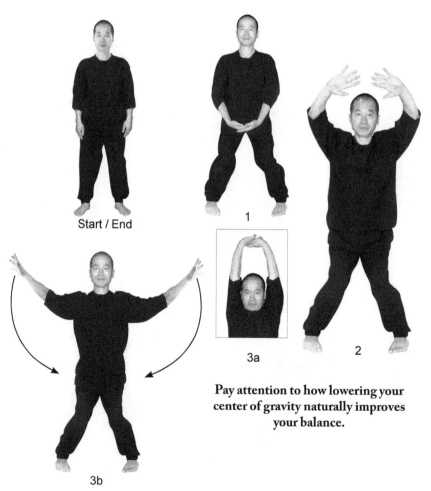

Start / End

1

3a

2

3b

Pay attention to how lowering your center of gravity naturally improves your balance.

Headache

Headaches are triggered by stress, a head injury, high blood pressure, a fever, a medical condition, food, or smells. Headache causes physical and mental tension, limits your ability to concentrate, and often debilitates your functional capacity. You can reduce the pain associated with a headache: by applying acupressure or by engaging in slow mindful movements that stimulate the appropriate meridians.

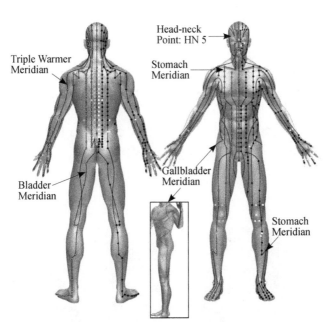

MERIDIANS FOR HEADACHE

Meridian	Accupoint	Exercise
Head-neck Points	HN 5	Acupressure
Bladder Meridian	BL 2, 10	Big Bow
Gallbladder Meridian	GB 20	Cradling
Stomach Meridian	ST 3	Infinity

Acupressure:

By gently pressing specific accupoints on the head and face, you can relieve many types of headaches. For optimal effect, gently press the point while exhaling. Increase the pressure gradually, using a long exhalation.

1. **HN 5 (temple):** Place the tip of your middle finger on the temple. Inhale. Close your eyes. Exhaling, gently press or massage the HN 5 point. Inhale and relax. Repeat this process until your headache is reduced.
2. **BL 2 (inner upper corner of the eye):** Place the tips of your thumbs upward on BL 2 point. Inhale. Close your eyes. Exhaling, gently press the point. Inhale and relax.
3. **BL 10 (rear neck):** Place the tip of your thumbs on both BL 10 points. Inhale. Close your eyes. Exhaling, gently press the points and increase pressure. Inhale and relax.
4. **GB 20 (rear neck):** Place the tip of your thumbs on GB 20 points. Inhale. Close your eyes. Exhaling, deeply press the points. Inhale and relax.
5. **ST 3 (middle cheek):** Place the tips of your middle fingers on ST 3 points. Inhale. Exhaling, gently press the points. Inhale and relax. Repeat this process until your headache is reduced.

HEADACHE

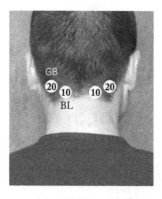
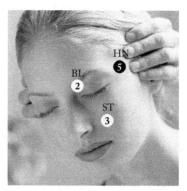

BIG BOW

1. From natural stance, inhaling, stretch your arms as high as you can with one hand overlapping the other and the palms facing upward.
2. Exhaling, slowly lower your stance.
3. Inhaling, slowly bend your body forward and reach your hands out to the front until your hands reach the floor (3a-3b).
4. Exhaling, lift your hip slightly and stretch your arms further forward (or place your hands on the floor). Feel the release in the lower back. This is the key movement in this posture to reduce a heavy sensation in the head.
5. Inhaling, very slowly arch your back and bring your body up to natural stance.

Big Bow posture facilitates energy flow from the bottom of the feet to the head and back to the feet, enhancing the circulation of blocked energy.

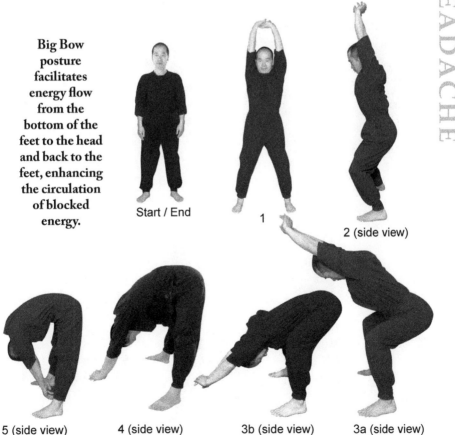

Start / End   1   2 (side view)

5 (side view)   4 (side view)   3b (side view)   3a (side view)

HEADACHE

CRADLING

1. From natural stance, place your arms around your body with your hands on the opposite tips of the shoulders. Inhale.
2. Exhaling, slowly turn your head to the left, and then turn your torso. Push your right leg toward your left leg for an additional twist. Hold that position for 3-5 seconds.
3. Inhaling, turn your body to the front.
4. Exhaling, slowly turn your head to the right, and then your torso. Push your left leg toward your right leg for an additional twist. Hold that position for 3-5 seconds.
5. Inhaling, turn your body to the front. Exhaling, return to natural stance.

HEADACHE

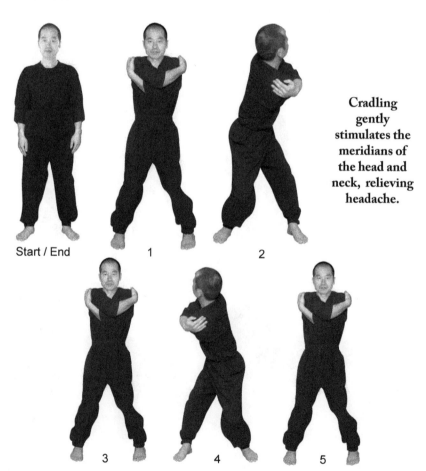

Cradling gently stimulates the meridians of the head and neck, relieving headache.

Start / End   1   2

3   4   5

INFINITY

1. From natural stance, point your heels outward and bend your knees. Place your open hands in front of your belly with palms facing upward. Exhale
2. Inhaling, raise your hands above your head with your fingers wide open. Pause for 3 seconds. Exhaling very slowly, bend your knees slightly. In the same position, inhale quickly and deeply; then exhale very slowly.
3. Inhaling deeply, push your hands upward to maximum extension (3a). Slowly exhale while lowering your hands sideways to your hips (3b). End in natural stance.

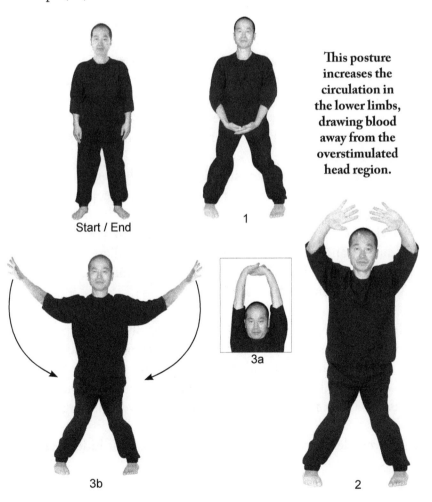

This posture increases the circulation in the lower limbs, drawing blood away from the overstimulated head region.

Start / End

1

3a

3b

2

HEADACHE

CONCLUSION

You have come to this point, exploring, discovering, and mastering what *the four pillars of MBX* encompass. At this juncture, your understanding should be deeper than when you began and will become deeper still as you practice. With that in mind, here are a few last words about each of the pillars to guide you to the next level:

1. **Mindfulness** is a manifestation of who you are as a result of your whole-hearted effort. Hindrance is reduced or annihilated in the face of your attainment of holistic awareness.
2. **Movement** awakens your senses, stimulating the inner life force, and allows you to exchange energy with the universe, integrating the two forces.
3. **Breath** connects the deepest cells in the body to the fathomless source of energy of the outer world. Breathe deeply, relax, and listen to the silence of your breath.
4. **Meridians** channel your energy according to your will. Your thoughts and intent alter the utility of meridians. Drive your energy through the 12 meridian circuits by mindful practice of MBX, for it builds the essential Ki.

Finally, the *three steps of mindful movement* should be practiced, without conscious effort, for each posture. **Attention** awakens your body and contains the mind. **Centering** brings energy from the upper energy center to the lower center, building your inner power. **Release** occurs at fullness and commences a new beginning.

These seven elements are the keys to mastering your hidden energy.

Meet Sang H. Kim

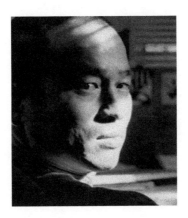

Sang H. Kim is the originator of MBX, mindful movement and deep breathing exercises. Dr. Kim is an internationally respected author of over 20 books on mindfulness, motivation, health, fitness, and martial arts, including *Ultimate Flexibility*, *Vital Point Strikes*, *Ultimate Fitness through Martial Arts*, *1001 Ways to Motivate Yourself and Others*, *Power Breathing*, *The Art of Harmony*, and *Martial Arts After 40*. He has also created over 200 instructional video programs on those subjects.

Dr. Kim has a PhD in Exercise Science, and had training as a Postdoctoral research fellow at the National Institutes of Health (NIH). He also had additional training at the National Cancer Institute (NCI) and the Institute of Lifestyle Medicine of Harvard Medical School.

He currently resides in the Washington, D.C. Metro area with his wife, Cynthia. He blogs at OneMindOneBreath.com.

Index

Symbols

3-3-6 breath cycle 50

A

Acceptance mudra 151
accupoint 63, 65, 100, 149, 174
acupressure 173–174
adenosine triphosphate 119
adrenalin 18
allostasis 18–19
allostatic overload 18–19
anxiety 79, 158–167
attention 11–14, 17, 19–21,
        24–25, 27–30, 32, 35–36,
        41–42, 46, 47, 59, 68, 76,
        82, 91, 106, 111, 124, 151,
        153, 164, 172
Attitude mudra 155
Awakening posture 44–47, 79
awareness 16, 20, 28, 42, 97,
        130, 168
Ayurveda 22

B

balance 17–19, 30, 40, 42, 57,
        69, 75, 83, 89, 92, 107,
        117, 132, 168–172
belly breathing 52, 120–121
Belt channel 53
Benevolence mudra 149
Big Bow posture 92–95, 96, 159
biorhythms 77
BL2 accupoint 174
BL 10 accupoint 174
Bladder Meridian 40, 88, 92, 94,
        100, 173
blood pressure 50, 79, 80, 84,
        90, 92, 158, 173

brain function 21–22, 86
breath control 120–121
breathing 20, 43, 50–53, 136
    deep 9, 13, 50, 84, 90, 97, 108,
        112, 119, 120, 128, 179
    mechanics 51
    techniques 52–53
Bubbling Spring 100
Buddha 112

C

Calm Hands mudra 153
Cannon, Walter 18
carbon dioxide 113
Carrier posture 54–57, 162–163
centering 13, 14, 25, 30, 35, 42,
        117, 132
Central energy flow 141,
        146–147, 150–151, 154
cerebellum 96
chest breathing 120–121
chi 22
chronic stress 91
circadian rhythm 77
circulation 57, 84, 86, 92, 101,
        109, 113, 116–118, 157,
        175, 177–178
circulatory system 84
compression posture 106
Conception meridian 53
Condensing posture 104–108
confidence 30
cortisol 18
Cradling posture 122–126, 169,
        176
Crane Stance 38

D

danjeon 63

dantien 63
Diamond Hands mudra 145
diaphragm 12, 23, 44, 47–48, 51, 52, 80, 83, 101, 104–108, 111, 114, 118, 120–121
diaphragm strengthening 104–105
digestion 66, 86, 118
dizziness 40, 86, 92, 116
double exhaling 136
double inhaling 136

E

Eastern Medicine 49, 63, 77, 85, 109, 141, 142
energy 16, 18
  centers 63, 65, 98
  efficiency 16
  essential 22
  explosive 110–111
  hubs 65
exterior meridians 34

F

Finger Wheel posture 72–75
five organs 64
fluidity 78
Forward bending postures 39
four pillars of energy transformation 9, 10, 35

G

Gallbladder Meridian 40, 116, 122, 124, 132
GB 20 accupoint 174
Goat Stance 38
Goose Head mudra 154
Governing meridian 53

H

headache 173–177

Heart Meridian 40, 74, 80, 82, 88, 148–149
heart rate 50, 79, 80, 90, 128, 178
Heavenly Fingers mudra 148
HN 5 accupoint 174
homeostasis 16–18
hormones 85
Horse Stance 31, 38, 125

I

immune system 85
Infinity posture 13, 31, 66–69, 79, 96, 161, 172, 177
Intelligence mudra 152
interior meridians 34
internal clock 77
interoception 16, 17, 21
interstitial fluid 70–71
Interwoven Fingers mudra 147
intestines 89

K

ki 22, 26, 159
  collection 103
  expressive 26, 61
  receptive 26, 59–61
  redistribution 103
kiai 110–111
Kidney Meridian 40, 94, 98, 100, 106, 158, 168
kidneys 98
kihap 110–111

L

Lao Tzu 26, 64
Large Intestine Meridian 40, 46, 54, 56–57, 68, 146–147
lifestyle change 90–91
Liver Meridian 40, 46, 124, 130, 132, 158

Lotus posture 96, 98–101, 160, 170
lower energy center 13, 62, 63, 65–66, 72, 80, 103, 109, 111, 132
lower warmer 114, 118
Loyalty mudra 150
lung 22
Lung Meridian 40, 44, 46, 48, 54, 56, 66, 72, 80, 104, 114, 122, 130, 132, 144, 145, 146, 150, 151
lymphatic channels 69, 70–71
lymphatic system 70–71

M

martial art 110–111
MBX 25–32
MBX-12 7–9, 34–40, 49, 77, 79, 90, 103, 130–134, 136–139, 141, 157
MBX-12 sequence. 35, 36, 134–139
meditation 19, 20, 21, 23–24, 85, 91
meridian 9, 10, 34, 40, 44, 45, 48, 53, 54, 77, 80, 118, 125, 142, 146–147, 149, 154–157, 159, 163, 178
  breathing 53
  cycle 49, 77
  yang 34, 53, 141
  yin 34, 53, 141
middle energy center 13, 62, 65–66, 72, 103, 105, 108–109, 132
middle warmer 114, 118
mind-body unity 127
mindful movement 25–32, 78, 84, 90, 102–103, 128
mindfulness 11–21, 151
modified child pose 40, 86
mudra 141–152

N

nasal breathing 112
natural stance 38
nervous system 128
neuroendocrine function 90, 128
nitric oxide 43, 84, 112, 113

O

oxygen 25, 43–44, 50, 84–85, 97, 111–113, 118–119, 121, 128

P

pain 14, 27
parasympathetic nervous system 41, 47, 79, 84, 90, 111, 128
Peacock posture 80–83
Pericardium Meridian 40, 100, 104, 106, 116, 152, 153
peripheral oscillators 77
piriformis muscle 132
Planting posture 114–117, 166–167
point of conception 63
posture 36, 39, 42
prana 22
proprioceptors 73, 96, 168

R

rear arching postures 39
Reflection mudra 156
release. 13, 25, 35, 111, 156
repetition 41
resistance 102–103
rhythm 42
rhythmic breathing 129

S

self-assessment criteria 41–42
self-confidence 30

self-regulation 47
sensory information 76
sleep 129
Small Intestine Meridian 40, 82,
    86, 88, 94, 150, 151
spleen 74
Spleen Meridian 40, 68, 72, 74,
    75, 82
ST 3 accupoint 174
stamina 98
stance 38
Stomach Meridian 37, 40, 56,
    66, 68, 74, 158, 168, 173
stress 79, 128
Stress resilience 90–91
suprachiasmatic nucleus 77
sympathetic nervous system 41,
    79, 90, 128

T

Taoism 26, 58
tension 32, 74, 83, 86, 89, 95,
    155
terminal energy flow 141,
    144–145, 148–149, 152
third eye 65
Thumbs Up mudra 144
torso twisting postures 39
Triad mudra 146, 147
Triple Warmer 8, 40, 106, 114,
    116, 118, 124, 142, 154,
    155
Triple Warmer Meridian 40, 106,
    114, 116, 124, 154–155
Twins posture 86–89, 171
twisting 69, 70–71, 114, 125

U

Unity posture 130–133, 164–165
upper energy center 65, 109, 132
upper warmer 114, 118

Upright postures 39

V

vagus nerve 79, 84, 90, 152
vasodilation 108, 128

W

warm-up 143
wringing 125

Y

yang 7, 26, 34, 53, 61, 141, 150,
    168, 173
  energy 61–63
yin 7, 26, 34, 53, 61, 63, 141,
    149, 153, 168, 173
  energy 61–63
yin-yang diagram 19, 61–62

CPSIA information can be obtained
at www.ICGtesting.com
Printed in the USA
BVHW031541191218
535965BV00009B/880/P